Arthroscopy of the Knee

Arthroscopy of the Knee

Reinhard Aigner and Jan Gillquist

with contributions by Karola Sommerlath and Martin Pilstl
Foreword by David Dandy

73 illustrations

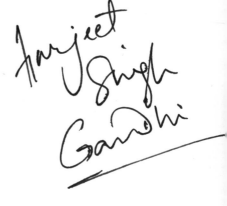

1991
Georg Thieme Verlag Stuttgart · New York
Thieme Medical Publishers, Inc., New York

Reinhard Aigner, M.D.
Schönfeldstr. 14, 8000 Munich 22
Federal Republic of Germany

Prof. Jan Gillquist, M.D.
University Orthopedic Clinic
Regional Hospital
58185 Linköping, Sweden

Martin Pilstl, M.D.
Schönfeldstr.14, 8000 Munich 22
Federal Republic of Germany

Karola Sommerlath, M.D.
University Orthopedic Clinic
Regional Hospital
58185 Linköping, Sweden

Translated by
Claus Röhrborn, M.D.
Division of Urology University of Texas
Southwestern Medical School
5323 Harry Hines Blvd.
Dallas, TX 75235-9031, USA

With the cooperation of Karl H. Mueller
Clinical Professor Emeritus Medical College of
Wisconsin Department of Orthopedic Surgery
2015 Hallyhock Lane
Elm Grove, WI 53122, USA

Illustrated by Martin Pilstl and Joachim Hormann

Cover design: D. Loenicker, Stuttgart

Deutsche Bibliothek Cataloguing in Publication Data

Aigner, Reinhard:
Arthroscopy of the Knee / Reinhard Aigner ; Jan Gillquist. With contributions by Karola
Sommerlath and Martin Pilstl. Foreword by David Dandy. [Transl. by Claus Röhrborn with
the cooperation of Karl H. Müller]. – Stuttgart ; New York : Thieme ; New York : Thieme
Med. Publ., 1991
    Dt. Ausg. u.d.T.: Aigner, Reinhard: Arthroskopie des Kniegelenks
NE: Gillquist, Jan:

Important Note: Medicine is an ever-changing science undergoing continual development. Research and clinical experience are continually expanding our knowledge, in
particular our knowledge of proper treatment and drug therapy. Insofar as this book
mentions any dosage or application, readers may rest assured that the authors, editors
and publishers have made every effort to ensure that such references are in accordance
with the state of knowledge at the time of production of the book. Nevertheless this does
not involve, imply, or express any guarantee or responsibility on the part of the publishers
in respect of any dosage instructions and forms of application stated in the book. Every
user is requested to examine carefully the manufacturers' leaflets accompanying each
drug and to check, if necessary in consultation with a physician or specialist, whether the
dosage schedules mentioned therein or the contraindications stated by the manufacturers
differ from the statements made in the present book. Such examination is particularly
important with drugs that are either rarely used or have been newly released on the
market. Every dosage schedule or every form of application used is entirely at the user's
own risk and responsibility. The authors and publishers request every user to report to the
publishers any discrepancies or inaccuracies noticed.

© 1991 Georg Thieme Verlag, Rüdigerstrasse 14, D-7000 Stuttgart 30, Germany
Thieme Medical Publishers, Inc., 381 Park Avenue South, New York, N.Y. 10016
Typesetting by Druckhaus Götz KG, Ludwigsburg (Linotron 202 [System 5])
Printed in Germany by Grammlich, Pliezhausen

ISBN 3-13-743201-4 (Georg Thieme Verlag, Stuttgart)
ISBN 0-86577-342-4 (Thieme Medical Publishers, Inc., New York)   1   2   3   4   5   6

Foreword

Fifteen years ago, arthroscopy of the knee was almost unheard of. Today, it is the most commonly performed orthopedic operation in many countries and continues to increase in popularity. Few techniques have had such an immediate impact on surgery or brought such enormous benefits to patients in such a short period.

This explosive development of arthroscopy has also created a number of problems. The anatomy of the knee had to be redefined, new instruments devised, new skills and operative techniques developed, and means found both to prevent and to treat complications not previously encountered. Inevitably, the earlier text books were incomplete and some of the techniques described therein have not stood the test of time.

It has taken over a decade for a consensus on arthroscopy of the knee to be reached and for the subject to consolidate. The time is now ripe for an authoritative text by experienced surgeons, and Doctors Aigner and Gillquist have provided exactly what was needed. Previous texts have been based on practice in North America, Europe, or the United Kingdom, but this narrow view has been overcome by these authors, who are able to draw upon practical experience in both the English-speaking and German-speaking worlds, in Scandinavia, North America, and Europe.

I have no doubt that this elegant and authoritative work will define the standard practice of arthroscopy of the knee around the world and become a classic reference work.

Cambridge, 1991   *David Dandy*

Preface

In this short book, we have tried to present the current status of
arthroscopy of the knee and its direction of development in the near
future. By choosing the paperback format, we hope to make this
information available not only to all interested physicians but also to
interns and students.

Arthroscopy is no longer a special technique; it has become an everyday
method. In the last two decades, clear ideas about indications and
methodology have developed.

While appreciating other methods currently being used, we would like
to present here a generally applicable procedure.

Munich and Linköping 1991   *Reinhard Aigner*
                                                     Jan Gillquist

Errata

Page 20, Fig. **12**: Illustrations **a–c** are in the wrong order.

   a should be **b**
   b should be **c**
   c should be **a**

Page 121: Fig. **94c** is inverted.

Aigner/Gillquist: Arthroscopy of the Knee
ISBN 3-13-743201-4
Georg Thieme Verlag Stuttgart · New York
8/91

Contents

Introduction 1

Anatomy of the Knee and Arthroscopy 3
    Complex Structure 3
    Synovial space 4
    Bony Structures 8
    Ligaments and Muscles 10
    Cruciate Ligaments 13
    Menisci 14
    Juxta-articular Structures 18
    Biomechanics of the Joint 19
Techniques and Prerequisites 22
    Synopsis of Prerequisites 22
    Choice of Procedure 22
    Selection of Anesthesia 23
    Selection of the Filling Medium 24
    Choice of Approach 29
    Selection of Instruments 32
    The Arthroscopic Operation 48
Problems and Complications 53
    Incidence 53
    Infection 53
    Fluid Leak 54
    Gas Leak 54
    Damage to Articular Cartilage 54
    General Risks 54
Indications, Contraindications and Alternative Methods 55
    Indications 55
    Contraindications 58
    Alternative Methods 59

Diagnostic Arthroscopy 60

Principles and Indications 60
Technique 60
    Approach to the Joint 60
    Examining the Joint Space 64
Examination of the Menisci 74
    Arthroscopic Diagnosis of the Menisci 75

Examination of Capsule and Ligaments 82
   Clinical Examination of Capsule and Ligaments 82
   Arthroscopic Evaluation of Capsular and Ligamentous
   Structures 83
Evaluation of Articular Cartilage and Patella 86
   Examination of Articular Cartilage 86
   Examination of the Patella 89
Disorders of the Synovial Membrane and Plica Syndrome 91
   Disorders of the Synovium 91
   Plica Syndrome 92
Arthroscopy in Acute Trauma 93
   Osteochondral Lesions 95
   Lesions of Ligaments and Menisci 96

Arthroscopic Surgery 98

Survey of Indications, Prerequisites, and Techniques 98
Meniscus Surgery 99
   Longitudinal Tear, Undisplaced Type 99
   Bucket Handle Tear 100
   Flap Tear 100
   Radial Tear 105
   Horizontal Tears 106
   Discoid Meniscus 108
   Meniscus Repair 108
   Posterior Joint Space 113
   Lost Fragment 115
   Summary of Important Steps in Meniscus Surgery 115
Surgery of the Joint Surfaces 116
   Surgery of the Cartilage 117
   Surgery of the Bone 118
   Surgery of the Synovium 120
   Loose Bodies 123
Arthroscopy and Miniarthrotomy 124
Replacement and Repair of the Cruciate Ligament 125

Documentation, Rehabilitation, and Late Results 128

Documentation 128
Rehabilitation 129
   Postoperative Care 129
   Exercise Program after Operative Arthroscopy of the Knee
   Joint 132
Late Results 136
References 139
Index 145

Introduction

Arthroscopy is well established as a method of endoscopic examination of joints in orthopedic surgery.

In principle, arthroscopy is suitable for any joint, whose joint space can be distended to a size which accommodates arthroscopic instruments, using reasonable intra-articular pressures by means of water, gas, or external traction. These include the knee joint, the shoulder joint as well as the hip joint. Indications for the wrist, elbow and ankle joints are limited to diagnostic procedures.

After initial trials more than 50 years ago* with most unsuitable cystoscopes and laparoscopes, the methodology has been further developed since 1970. Prerequisites for this progress were adequate optical systems, light guides and light sources. Modern video technology provided further advances. Today, a stage of consolidation has been reached, after passing through the stages of original idea, realization, improvement and widespread usage.

By combining different approaches, a more or less uniform technique of arthroscopy has now been developed.

Diagnostic arthroscopy opens new possibilities for the evaluation of long-standing joint problems which continue to recur despite intensive treatment. In many cases, a thorough clinical workup results in arthroscopic or open surgery. Diagnostic arthroscopy can be extended into an arthroscopic operation. Traumatic lesions of articular cartilage, which were often difficult to diagnose in the past, can now be demonstrated and treated. The diagnosis of different types of metaplastic changes of the synovium and various rheumatic diseases is made much easier by arthroscopy.

Diagnostic arthroscopy has developed into arthroscopic surgery in the meantime, with the same indications that apply to conventional arthrotomy.

The advantages of arthroscopic surgery are obvious: small incisions, a shorter hospital stay, and a shorter rehabilitation period.

The main advantage conventional arthrotomy seems to offer, namely a wide-open operative field, is frequently overrated by the orthopedic

---

* *Historical note.* 1918, arthroscopy of the knee joint by Takagi with a cystoscope; 1920, by Bircher with a laparoscope, 1920 by Takagi with an arthroscope.

surgeon not used to arthroscopy. Only arthroscopy allows visualization of all joint compartments.

We have developed a method by which the entire joint space can be viewed with the optical system of a rigid arthroscope through an incision in the patellar tendon. While the posterior horn of the meniscus can not be visualized with conventional arthrotomy, the angled lens of the modern arthroscope allows inspection of the meniscus and possible lesions can be detected with the probing hook.

Arthroscopic procedures for removal of loose bodies, repair of cartilage lesions, for lateral release of the patella as well as removal of damaged menisci have become routine operations in many institutions.

In arthroscopy centers, surgical procedures are usually videotaped which assists in resident teaching and allows accurate documentation.

Motorized instruments have now been developed to facilitate arthroscopic surgery and to save time. Arthroscopic electroresection is another recent advance.

With this new technology, arthroscopy can be used for more extensive surgical procedures, for example, replacement of the anterior cruciate ligament, debridement of joints with degenerative changes and total synovectomy.

Reattachment of a torn meniscus, if intraoperative findings warrant it, has become a routine operation.

Indications for arthroscopy have changed considerably during the last 20 years; 80% of all arthroscopies are surgical procedures today, while in the past, 80% were done for diagnostic purposes.

When used appropriately, the method affords significant advantages for the patient and offers better visualization of the joint space.

However, inadequate training and the inexperience of the beginner constitute a certain risk, and we believe that arthroscopy should be performed only in institutions with adequate expertise in the surgical treatment of joint disorders.

Arthroscopy is a special surgical technique which can only be taught and learned directly, individually and step by step (Fig. **1**). Consequently, the first step should be diagnostic arthroscopy, followed by arthroscopic biopsy, removal of loose bodies, arthroscopic meniscectomy, removal of bucket handle tears and finally synovectomy. Special courses are offered to teach the necessary skills to the beginner and to resolve the questions and problems the more advanced arthroscopist may have. Fortunately, the same tools, namely videotapes, can be used for teaching and in the operating room.

Several groups have been formed worldwide for the exchange of ideas, experience, and results, and numerous journals and special publications are available (see references). The International Arthroscopy Association (IAA) has been in existence for several years and holds a major meeting every second year together with the International Society of the

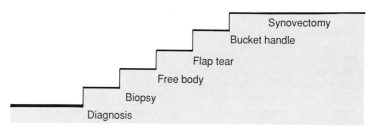

Fig. 1 Stepladder for teaching and continuing education in arthroscopy. Simple diagnostic procedures, biopsies, etc., should be performed first before major surgical procedures, for example, removal of a degenerated posterior meniscus horn, are attempted (after Dandy)

Knee (ISK) with the purpose of exchanging experiences and introducing new techniques concerning the arthroscopy of different joints. Normally, an international course is held in the year between meetings. In German-speaking countries, the Association of German-speaking Arthroscopists (AGA), as well as other associations have been founded for the same reasons, for example, the Arthroscopy Association of North America (AANA). Many journals are now available which mainly publish papers concerning arthroscopy such as the Journal of Arthroscopy, and the Zeitschrift für Arthroskopie. The quality of instruction is not determined by the location of the teaching institution but by the enthusiasm and experience of the individual teachers.

This introduction is intended to make our experience available to interested students and physicians.

Furthermore, it should help the more advanced arthroscopist to fulfill the following requirements:

- rapid and logical inspection of the entire joint space;
- orientation within the joint and recognition of pathological conditions;
- complete but simple equipment to save time, money, and personnel.

Anatomy of the Knee and Arthroscopy

Complex Structure

The complexity of the largest joint in the human body, the knee joint, results not only in a high vulnerability to injury, but also in a high degree of difficulty in assessing damage to it. While on the surface the complexity of form and structure offers an easy explanation for this problem, nevertheless, an accurate diagnosis remains very difficult to establish, even after exact analysis of all elements forming the knee and all its possible movements.

One aspect becomes clear in the so-called "law of the ligaments" as formulated by Sir Arthur Keith 60 years ago: "At the knee, ligaments limit and control the articular surface at all stages of movement, but at no stage are the ligaments left without the active support of muscular action." The ligaments, which are only looked upon as static guidelines during reconstruction, are, especially in the knee, always supported by active muscular elements. At the level of the joint space the tendon attachments are combined with the collateral and cruciate ligaments to form common structures which facilitate arthroscopy on the one hand and allow entrance into the joint on the other hand (for example, central approach through the patellar tendon).

Arthroscopic anatomy is mainly surface-oriented. Synovium, cruciate ligaments, and menisci, as well as the articular cartilage surfaces and the undersurface of the patella, are of particular importance.

Synovial space

Arthroscopic operations, visualization as well as movements, are restricted to the space created by expanding the joint under pressure. This space depends on the position of the joint. It is surrounded by synovial membrane, articular cartilage, and menisci (Fig. 2).

The joint space lined by the synovial membrane is variable. Joint surfaces of the knee are not congruent; the menisci interrupt the synovial membrane laterally. The wide range of motion of the knee in flexion and extension has caused the development of large recessus (Fig. 3). Cartilage surfaces and menisci are not covered by synovium. However, the cruciate ligaments (Fig. 4) and the popliteal tendon, which traverse the joint space, and the popliteal tendon in the hiatus popliteus of the lateral meniscus have a synovial sheath.

The so-called plicae are special structures which are derived from the synovial membrane. The superior recess (suprapatellar pouch) is variable; a classification of the variations is not worthwhile. Bridle-like plicae are present on both sides of the patella. A medial parapatellar plica is very common and can cause a pathological rubbing phenomenon on the articular cartilage of the medial femoral condyle.

The ligamentum mucosum (plica infrapatellaris) is regularly present (Fig. 5). The beginner frequently confuses it with the anterior cruciate ligament which runs almost parallel with it. This plica occasionally makes it difficult to change from one compartment to another. It is of no importance and can be resected if necessary.

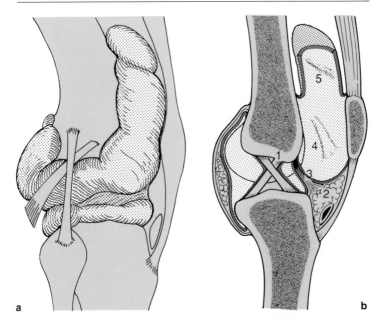

Fig. **2** The volume of the joint space is approximately 100 ml in the healthy knee. It is surrounded by a synovial membrane, articular cartilage, and the menisci. On the anterior aspect of the femur, it extends far cranially; the surfaces lined by synovial membrane are interrupted by the menisci (**a**).

The sagittal cut at the mid-patellar level (**b**) shows parts of the intra-articular structures: 1) cruciate ligaments, 2) Hoffa's fat pad, 3) ligamentum mucosum, 4) plica synovialis mediopatellaris, 5) superior recess

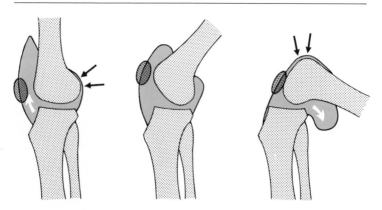

Fig. 3 If an effusion is present, the joint space widens during extension toward the suprapatellar pouch under the influence of the pressure from the quadriceps muscle. During flexion it expands into the popliteal fossa. This space is at its largest during 30° flexion, which is the reason that the knee with painful swelling and effusion is usually held in a position of 30° of flexion (drawing after Kapandji)

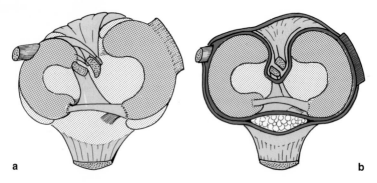

Fig. 4 The tibial plateau from above. For this and all following figures, the arthroscopic viewpoint is used (anterior structures are at the bottom in the drawings). Menisci and cruciate ligaments as the internal structures of the knee joint are connected by connective tissue at their ends (a). The two cruciate ligaments habe a common synovial sheath (b). This is of particular importance for the diagnosis of a rupture, as the synovial lining may cover up ruptured fibers (Fig. 67)

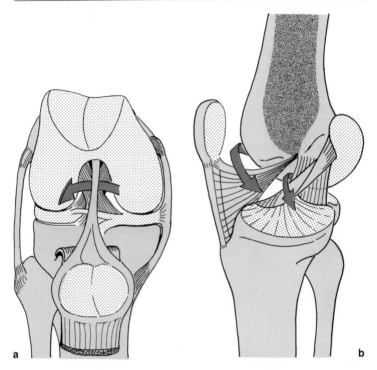

a   b

Fig. 5 The ligamentum mucosum. The medial and lateral compartments of the knee joint are separated by the common synovial sheath of the cruciate ligaments on one side and by the ligamentum mucosum on the other side. In passing the arthroscope from the inner to the outer joint space, this can represent an obstruction as well as a possibility for confusion with the anterior cruciate ligament. If the direct route in changing from one compartment to another is not possible, the ligamentum mucosum has to be circumvented by following the edge of the cartilage in the intracondylar notch (drawings after Kapandji)

Bony Structures

The bony elements which form the static basis of the knee joint have very incongruent surfaces. Congruity between the surfaces is established by connective tissue structures. The femoral condyles are two round, eccentrically curved protruberances with an anterior oval and a posterior spherical shape. They form the intercondylar notch between them, which contains the cruciate ligaments. The trochlear groove lies anteriorly betwen the two condyles and forms the gliding path for the patella when the knee moves in flexion and extension. These bony structures can be demonstrated by conventional X-rays in preparation for arthroscopy (Fig. **6**).

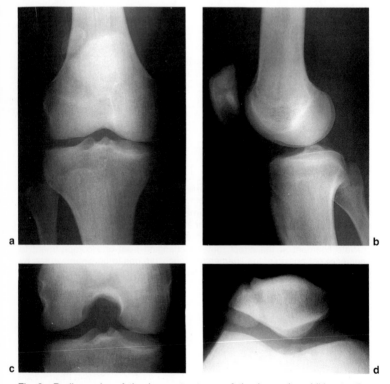

Fig. **6** Radiographs of the bony structures of the knee. In addition to the standard projections (anterior–posterior and lateral views: **a, b**), a tunnel view (Frik's view, **c**) and a tangential view of the patella (**d**) are routine parts of the radiological work-up prior to arthroscopy

The tibia articulates with the femoral condyles through two separate, flat plateaus. The tibial plateaus are separated by the eminentia inter-condylaris with a medial and lateral tibial spine. The menisci and the cruciate ligaments originate from areas in front of and behind the tibial spines. The joint surface of the medial tibial plateau is concave while the

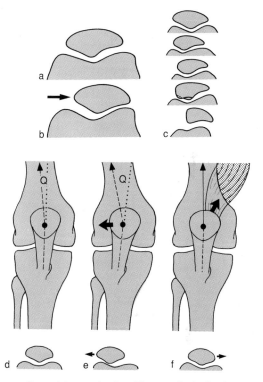

Fig. 7 The patella and its mechanics. The patella is the largest sesamoid bone of the human body. It has two large tendon insertions and its posterior surface is covered with articular cartilage. The articular surfaces of femur and patella are congruent during the first 30° of motion (**a**). Marked incongruence or lateralization (**b**) can cause clinical symptoms. Wiberg, as well as others, have classified the shape of the patella into five categories (**c**). Gait characteristics can be determined by the shape of the patella. The Q-angle (**d, e**) is the angle between the weight-bearing axis and the main direction of the extensor muscle pull; it is the biomechanical expression for the tendency of the patella to deviate laterally. The normal Q-angle ist 6°; if it is more than 12°, pathological gait characteristics can be expected. Alignment can be improved (**f**) by reinforcing the vastus medialis muscle

surface of the lateral plateau is slightly convex. Posteriorly, the lateral plateau drops off sharply; its articular cartilage continues beyond the posterior edge. When the meniscus is pulled back by the popliteal muscle, it glides backwards on this layer. Topography and contour of the lateral tibial plateau are probably of some importance for the mechanics of anterolateral rotatory stability ("pivot shift").

If the anterior cruciate ligament is insufficient, the lateral femoral condyle can slide backward and is probably trapped there for a short time until it may be brought back by contraction of the iliotibial band.

The patella (Fig. **7**) is a triangular-shaped and rounded sesamoid bone of the quadriceps muscle and its tendinous insertion and articulates with the trochlear groove, described above, provided femur and patella are congruent. If there is malalignment between the femoral and the tibial axis (increased valgus deformity) including a large Q-angle, patellofemoral symptoms may occur, especially if combined with a tilting or dysplasia of the patella itself, or both. The undersurface of the patella is covered by cartilage. A central protuberance on the undersurface corresponds with the trochlear groove. Different forms of patella are described, and a close connection between the form of the femur, the shape of the patella, as well as lateral guiding structures by the retinacula and muscle tracts can be defined arthroscopically.

Ligaments and Muscles

The knee joint is surrounded by a connective tissue envelope (the true joint capsule), as well as ligaments and tendons which cross the joint. The capsule is derived from these structures and forms a complete envelope for the knee joint (Fig. **8**).

This capsule has a substantial window in its anterior part, which is traversed by the extensor mechanism. All parts of the quadriceps muscle join in the patella to form the patellar tendon which extends to the lower part of the tibial tubercle. The patellar tendon and the palpable indentations at the joint space permit good arthroscopic orientation. Depending on the degree of flexion of the knee, the joint space opens (flexion) or closes (extension) anteriorly.

The medial structures can be divided into three parts. The anterior third extends from the medial border of the patella posteriorly to the anterior margin of the superficial medial collateral ligament and encloses the anteromedial retinaculum and the underlying capsule. The middle third consists of the superficial tibial collateral ligament and the underlying capsule which forms a capsular ligament here. The posterior third extends from the medial collateral ligament posteriorly to the posterior capsule and forms a sling over the medial femoral condyle. These fibers are under tension during extension of the knee and relax with flexion (Fig. **8c**).

The structures which provide medial stability are listed in Table **1**.
The lateral complex, like that of the medial side, consists of static and dynamic stabilizing elements (Table **2**; Fig. **8a**).
The lateral collateral ligament is a relatively short structure that extends from the lateral femoral condyle to the head of the fibula.
Mechanical tests have shown that this ligament is the primary restraint, resisting varus deformity of the knee together with the iliotibial band, the popliteal muscle, and the branches of the biceps tendon.

Table **1**   Stabilizing structures on the medial side oft the knee joint

Connective tissue (static)	Muscles (dynamic)
1. Capsule	1. Vastus medialis muscle
2. Medial collateral ligament	2. Muscles of the pes anserinus
3. Cruciate ligaments	3. Semimembranous muscle
4. Medial meniscus	4. Gastrocnemius muscle

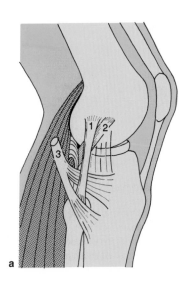
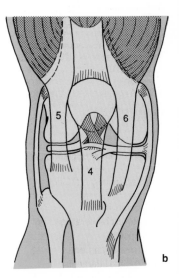

Fig. **8**   Muscles and ligaments of the knee joint. On the lateral side (**a**), the easily palpable lateral collateral ligament (1) allows good orientation. The popliteal muscle (2) and the biceps tendon (3) are crossing structures. The anterior side (**b**) is dominated by the patellar tendon (4), the capsular ligaments, and the extensor apparatus, which includes the lateral supporting ligaments (retinacula of the patella [5, 6]).

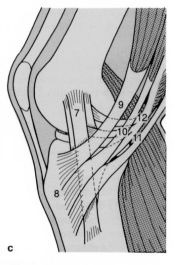 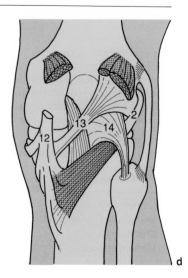

c   d

(Fig. **8** continue)
The medial collateral ligament with its double layer (7) and the pes anserinus (8) are visible on the medial side (**c**).
The semimembranous muscle (12) is hidden behind the three muscles forming the pes anserinus: the sartorius (9), gracilis (10), and semitendinosus (11) muscles. After removal of the large heads of the gastrocnemius muscle, the insertion of the semimembranous muscle is seen posteriorly (**d**), as well as the oblique ligament (13), the popliteal muscle (2) and the arcuate ligament (14)

Table **2**   Stabilizing structures on the lateral side of the knee joint

Connective tissue (static)	Muscles (dynamic)
1. Iliotibial band	1. Biceps femoris muscle
2. Lateral collateral ligament	2. Popliteal muscle
3. Capsule	3. Gastrocnemius muscle
4. Arcuate ligament	4. Vastus lateralis muscle
5. Cruciate ligaments	
6. Lateral meniscus	

In clinical practice the ligament can be easily demonstrated by having the patient place his or her leg over the opposite knee and drop the ipsilateral hip (Figure 4 position). This movement results in a varus stress on the knee during which the lateral collateral ligament can be easily palpated.

The structures of the posterior aspect of the knee joint are (Fig. **8 d**):

1. The posterior capsule,
2. The oblique popliteal ligament,
3. The arcuate ligament,
4. The popliteal muscle,
5. The tendons of the gastrocnemius muscle.

The popliteal muscle is located on the posterior surface of the tibia. It runs in an oblique fashion in a proximal and lateral direction with its tendinous origin. The medial two thirds of the muscle insert at the arcuate ligament and the posterior part of the lateral meniscus, while the lateral part becomes a tendon which runs alongside the femoral condyle under the lateral collateral ligament and inserts at the femoral condyle. The popliteal muscle is primarily an internal rotator of the tibia in relation to the femur, but it also prevents forward sliding of the femur on the tibia during flexion of the knee. During normal walking, the popliteal muscle becomes activated in the middle of the swing phase.

Cruciate Ligaments

The anterior cruciate ligament originates from the lateral femoral condyle far posteriorly, close to the posterior limits of the knee joint, and extends in an anterior–inferior and medial direction to the inter-condylar eminence of the tibia (Fig. **4 a**). The stronger posterior cruciate ligament is located immediately behind the anterior cruciate ligament. It originates deep in the intercondylar notch from the lateral side of the medial femoral condyle and attaches to the posterior edge of the tibial plateau. These four insertion sites of the cruciate ligaments play an important role in diagnosis and reconstruction of cruciate ligament lesions.

The cruciate ligaments are located intra-articularly but outside the synovial membrane. Together they form the most important stabilizing mechanism of the knee joint (Fig. **4 b**).

It is important to remember that the anterior cruciate ligament is covered by a thin synovial layer. If this synovial layer remains intact after an injury, the ligament may appear normal (Fig. **67**). The synovial sheath must be split to allow observation of the ligament during the drawer test.

The special architecture of the cruciate ligaments makes their recon-struction and the development of artificial ligaments extremely difficult.

Despite their important stabilizing function for the knee, the cruciate ligaments are not well positioned to resist rotatory, varus or valgus stress. They are much better at resisting forces acting in an anterior or posterior direction. Their special function is difficult to describe, as they cannot be separated from the remainder of the ligamentous apparatus of the knee joint. The anterior cruciate ligament stabilizes the tibia against an anterior drawer. Clinical studies suggest, however, that the anterior drawer test may be negative even in the absence of the anterior cruciate ligament if the remaining ligaments are intact.

Menisci

One hundred years ago, Hueter postulated that the knowledge of normal and pathological function of the menisci would be of special importance for the practicing physician. In the largest joint of the human body, articulating surfaces, ligaments and muscles together with the menisci form a locomotor system which is a well-functioning unit despite the obvious incongruity of its articulating surfaces (Fig. **4a**).

The biomechanical function of the menisci appears to be that of shock absorption. They are shaped to conform to the femoral and tibial joint surfaces, to improve the congruity of the joint, and to enlarge the contact surfaces. They transmit pressure equally across the weight-bearing areas, and their special shape enhances anterior–posterior as well as medial–lateral stability.

In an otherwise intact knee, the loss of a meniscus has very little influence in an anterior–posterior direction, initially. Removal of the menisci and transsection of the cruciate ligaments causes significant anterior–posterior as well as rotatory instability. One can conclude from this that the menisci play an important role in preventing instability after loss of the cruciate ligaments. Therefore, absence of the cruciate ligaments usually leads to a deterioration of the menisci.

The articular cartilage and the underlying bony lamellae react like a ping-pong ball when contact is made with a hard surface (model for the knee joint without menisci): impression when contact is made, followed by a cushioning effect and vibrations. Although the respective areas of the meniscus are relatively thin, the cartilage reacts like a shock absorber after the initial hard contact by decreasing deformation energy in the periphery of the meniscus. The development of osteoarthritic changes after meniscectomy proves that shock absorption is inadequate after loss of the meniscus.

The increase in congruity is closely linked to the stability of the knee joint. Studies by the Weber brothers (1836) have shown that the femoral condyles perform a rolling and gliding motion which begins as a pure rolling motion and gradually transforms into a pure gliding motion. The transition from one motion into the other is determined by the anterior cruciate ligament and is different for both condyles: the medial condyle begins its gliding motion at 10° of flexion while the lateral condyle continues its rolling motion until knee flexion is 20° and then starts its gliding motion. Gliding motion in extreme flexion is limited by the posterior cruciate ligament.

The menisci follow all movements of the femoral condyles. During external rotation, the lateral meniscus moves anteriorly and the medial meniscus posteriorly while its edge moves further away from the joint space. With increasing flexion, the menisci move more and more posteriorly, being actively pulled by the semimembranous and popliteal muscles. The menisceal bodies are broadened and deformed.

Normal function of the menisci requires healthy cartilage tissue, normal arterial blood supply, and intact muscles. A circular vascular system originating from the popliteal artery surrounds the outer diameter of both menisci within the joint capsule. Collaterals exist to the vessels supplying the anterior and posterior cruciate ligaments. In particular, the insertion sites of the anterior and posterior horns are well vascularized (Fig. **9a**).

The vascular supply to the menisci is organized similarly to the arterial arcades in the bowel: arcuate arteries send radial vessels into the meniscus, which then either run radially or continue in an arcuate fashion (Fig. **9b**). The schematic cross-section shows the two different zones of the meniscus: the inner central zone, which is avascular and carries most of the pressure load, and the outer zone, with much better vascularity. The center of the meniscus contains a round area with the poorest vascular supply (Fig. **9c**). Diffusion from the surface and from the better-vascularized parts is poorest in this area. Because of the degenerative changes found here, it is drawn as a structure consisting of many bubbles. Meniscectomy should be performed outside the areas which are most prone to degeneration, thereby eliminating those parts of the meniscus in which cracks can develop, while the well-vascularized and important stabilizing elements of the menisci are left intact. This is particularly obvious in the lateral meniscus just behind the hiatus popliteus, which has a predilection for developing ganglions, which are much more common on the lateral side. Degenerative swelling is followed by mucoid degeneration and finally, a process comparable to the herniation of an intervertebral disk, namely the protrusion of a structure which is called ganglion.

The distribution of the total load acting on the joint over a larger surface and two different levels results in better lubrication by synovial fluid. The importance of this effect can only be estimated. It can be assumed that the mere presence of the menisci resulting in the displacement of synovial fluid to the appropriate places plays an important role in itself. This space-occupying effect also prevents synovial folds from being trapped between the articulating joint surfaces.

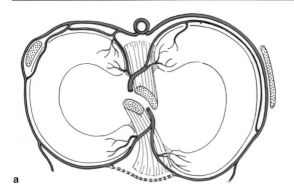

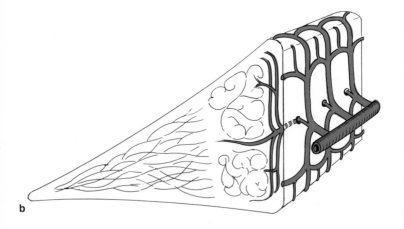

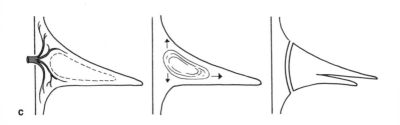

The menisci reduce extreme function in extension and thus prevent direct contact between cartilage-covered surfaces. They also prevent abrupt stress on the cruciate ligaments.

Follow-up examinations after meniscectomy have shown that degenerative changes develop in the knee joint in up to 75% of all cases, while only 6% of the patients had similar changes on the contralateral side. Meniscectomy reduces the ability to absorb energy and causes an increase in point-shaped contact areas. The total load remains approximately the same after meniscectomy, however, the contact surface is reduced significantly, and pressure per unit area is consequently more than doubled.

It is the prevailing opinion today, that the base of the meniscus has an important stabilizing function (brake-shoe effect), and the peripheral rim must be left in place after conservative arthroscopic meniscectomy (Figs. **10, 11**).

The microscopic architecture of the cartilage fibers is an important characteristic of the healthy meniscus. Fibers are arranged longitudinally and form intertwined arcades directed toward the tip of the meniscus according to a biological principle that exposes the circumference to greater traction forces when the meniscus is under compression.

A meniscus damaged by disease or trauma develops degenerative changes with fibrillation and swelling of the fibers and fibrillar degeneration of the connective tissue elements typical for cartilage. Reparative and proliferative processes manifest themselves as densely packed fibrocytes and pannus formation. Initially, the cells are arranged as individual cell foci; later, they involve the entire meniscus. Early stages of age-dependent degenerative changes develop at the end of the fourth decade of life and increase gradually to a moderate degree until the seventh decade.

These age-dependent primary degenerative changes vary significantly from one individual to the next. With individual disposition or chronic abuse through work-related or athletic activities, or both, degenerative processes may begin relatively early.

◀ Fig. **9**   Blood supply of the meniscus. The knee is surrounded by an arterial arcade which originates from the popliteal artery (**a**) and supplies the peripheral parts of the meniscus through radial arteries (**b**). Away from the capsule, the meniscus derives its nutrition by diffusion from the synovial fluid. The cross-section of the meniscus (**c**) shows how small structural disorders originating from the avascular central area can develop into horizontal and vertical tears (Fig. **61**)

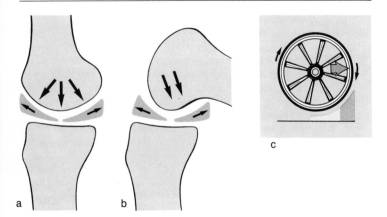

Fig. **10**   The function of the meniscus consists of the cushioning of axial forces and slowing tangential shearing forces.
a The axial forces are distributed over the meniscus onto the circular fibers of the meniscus base and the joint capsule.
b During extreme flexion and extension, the edge of the meniscus is fixed to the capsule and prevents direct contact between the articulating surfaces of tibia and femur.
c After partial meniscectomy, the remainder of the meniscus is still an important stabilizing and biomechanical element (brake-shoe function)

Total meniscectomy—which was done frequently and often unnecessarily in the past—regularly leads to further degenerative changes.
Osteoarthritic changes must be expected in 50−70% of all knee joints following total meniscectomy.

Juxta-articular Structures

When planning the arthroscopic approach, one must be careful not to enter the joint at sites where vital structures can be damaged when the joint is punctured or where the opposite wall of the capsule can be damaged when the instrument is advanced.
Juxta-articular structures "at risk" are illustrated in Figure **12.** The neurovascular bundle of the popliteal area is of primary importance. It is near the posterior capsule and could be damaged from the central approach, especially when the lance is extended. With increased flexion

Fig. **11**   Pressure distribution in the knee joint after meniscectomy (schematic). After removal of the meniscus a small zone of high pressure develops (large arrow). Together with other factors, progressive damage of the joint begins from here

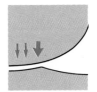

of the knee, these structures move further away from the joint space. Laterally, the peroneal nerve (fibular nerve) passes around the neck of the fibula. The nerve may be "at risk" with a lateral approach and also with a possible tibial compartment syndrome. On the medial side, the infrapatellar branch of the saphenous nerve and the saphenous vein can be damaged by inappropriate perforation.

Biomechanics of the Joint

Motion of the normal knee joint occurs around several different axes following biomechanical laws which can change when stability of the joint is abnormal. Figure **13** summarizes these mechanisms for the normal knee as far as the arthroscopically visible joint is concerned.

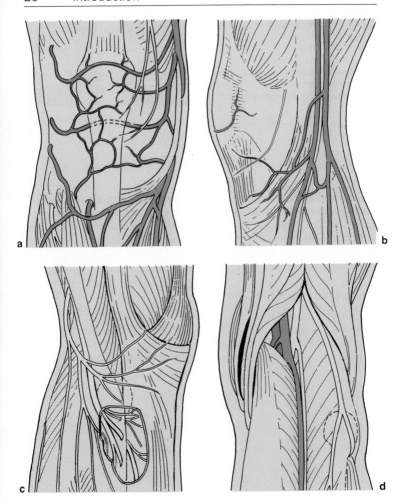

Fig. **12** Juxta-articular structures of importance for arthroscopic approaches and maneuvers.
a On the lateral side, the peroneal nerve must be protected.
b Anteriorly, damage to the infrapatellar nerve can result in sensory changes in an area below the patella.
c Medially, the saphenous vein (s) have to be avoided by careful introduction of the instruments in the posterior approach.
d The posterior structures of the popliteal fossa are also endangered through instruments introduced through other portals. A posterior approach is contraindicated

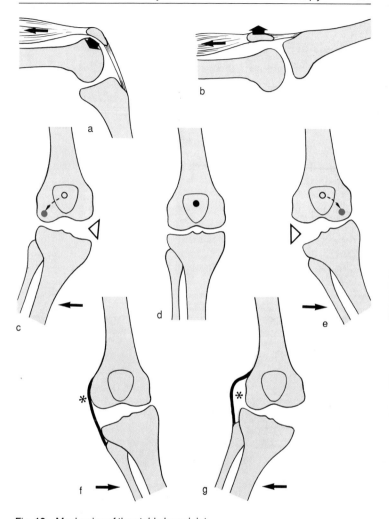

Fig. **13** Mechanics of the stable knee joint.
a, b Pressure of the patella against the femur is lowest or even negative when the knee is in extension. The arthroscope can be introduced best in this position.

c–e The varus–valgus axis of the medial and lateral joint components shifts during varus–valgus stress toward the center of the corresponding femoral condyle, especially in an unstable knee. The collateral ligament relaxes during valgus stress (paradoxical) and permits visualization of the lateral gutter (**f, g**)

Techniques and Prerequisites

Synopsis of Prerequisites

There is general agreement today regarding the methodology of arthroscopic surgery.

- Under general or regional anesthesia, even extensive and prolonged surgical procedures with multiple incisions can be performed.
- Liquid media and the application of a tourniquet allow good visualization and continuous irrigation of the distended joint.
- The use of video equipment provides the prerequisites for a sterile work place (Figs. **14, 15**), as well as offering advantages in teaching and documentation.

Choice of Procedure

Arthroscopy can be performed in many different ways. It can be done as a purely diagnostic procedure on an outpatient basis under local anesthesia and with gas insufflation of the joint. More extensive diag-

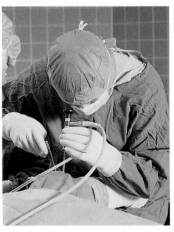 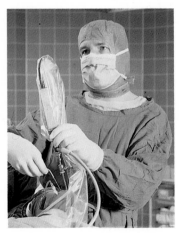

Fig. **14**   Fig. **15**

Fig. **14** Diagnostic arthroscopy can be performed under direct vision through the arthroscope

Fig. **15** For more involved procedures, a video system, which is easy to use and allows work under sterile conditions, should be used

Table **3**   Suitable methods for diagnostic and surgical arthroscopy of the knee joint

	Diagnostic Arthroscopy	Surgical Arthroscopy
Anesthesia	Local	General
Distension medium	Gas (CO_2)	Isotonic solutions
Approach	Anteromedial	Central

nostic procedures and arthroscopic surgery, on the other hand, should be done under general anesthesia in the operating theater using a liquid medium for distention and irrigation of the joint. All surgical procedures should be done under strictly aseptic conditions. We perform all knee operations with the highest degree of sterile technique and try to keep technical errors caused by arthroscopy equipment to a minimum.

With growing experience, we have been able to develop a clear and practical selection of procedures. For example, gas insufflation makes the necessary, intermittent irrigation of the joint during arthroscopic surgery more cumbersome, and a pain-free central approach is difficult to maintain under local anesthesia. These and other considerations have led us to the choice of methods listed in Table **3**.

The operative procedure is determined by the following criteria:

1. choice of anesthesia,
2. choice of filling medium,
3. choice of approach,
4. choice of instruments.

As these decisions can be complicated, they are discussed individually in the following paragraphs.

Selection of Anesthesia

Diagnostic arthroscopy can be performed under local anesthesia, thereby eliminating the need for general or regional anesthesia and postanesthesia recovery time. Diagnostic arthroscopy can be done on an outpatient basis.

However, local anesthesia has significant limitations in diagnostic arthroscopy, because certain phenomena which may interfere with the procedure cannot be eliminated during local anesthesia. Various pathological conditions, such as compartment blockage caused by a bucket handle tear or extensive adhesions (fibrosis of Hoffa's fat pad or the joint capsule, intra-articular adhesions or extensive synovitis), can make arthroscopic examination very difficult or even impossible. In addition, optimal visualization of the entire joint space cannot be obtained under local anesthesia. For diagnostic arthroscopy, the instrument is usually introduced anteromedially or anterolaterally, occasionally through a suprapatellar or a parapatellar approach, but very rarely posterome-dially or posterolaterally. Local anesthesia is not sufficient to allow introduction of the arthroscope through the patellar tendon; conse-quently, the approach which allows optimal visualization of the entire knee joint cannot be used with local anesthesia.

The posteromedial recessus (where debris usually collects), and the posterior cruciate ligament can not be visualized. Therefore, local anesthesia should be reserved for arthroscopy with purely diagnostic indications or synovial biopsies and should not be used for surgical procedures.

Arthroscopic surgery requires regional or general anesthesia. This pro-duces better muscle relaxation which makes the operation easier, facilitates separation of the joint surfaces, and allows the use of leg holders, a tourniquet, and a perfusion pump.

The main argument for general anesthesia is the possibility to use the central approach, which allows much better visualization of the joint space, and it leaves the other portals available for instruments.

Acute arthroscopy, for example, for a fresh post-traumatic hemarthro-sis, should be done under general anesthesia. This eliminates pain for the patient and permits arthrotomy for definitive repair of capsule and ligament tears, or lesions of meniscus and articular cartilage, or both, if they should be necessary.

Selection of the Filling Medium

Distention of the joint space with a gas or liquid medium is absolutely essential. It provides the necessary visualization, and can be used for atraumatic lysis of adhesions.

Historically, arthroscopy has been closely connected with gas insuffla-tion of the joint. The steady increase of operative procedures has made the transition from gas to liquid media necessary. Liquid media permit irrigation of the joint with removal of small hemorrhages and debris and provide constant, clear visualization.

Gas Insufflation

Several appliances are available which allow expansion of the joint by insufflation of gas through a pressure-reduction system with a filter for bacteria. This procedure provides excellent optical resolution for inspection and palpation of the joint, and it is the preferred medium for photography (Fig. **16**). Unfortunately, the high optical transparency of

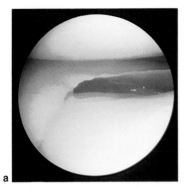 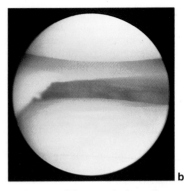

a   b

Fig. **16** Comparison between gas (**a**) and water (**b**) as optical medium. Visualization with gas insufflation is more brilliant under otherwise similar conditions

gas is useful only under ideal conditions. A surgical procedure which may be untertaken as a result of diagnostic arthrostic arthroscopy can be made difficult by bleeding, formation of bubbles, dirty lenses, debris, as well as an occasional gas emphysema.

At the beginning of and during the operative procedure, it is necessary to irrigate the joint frequently to remove particles. For outpatient diagnostic arthroscopy under local anesthesia, the gas insufflation method can be used successfully.

Unfortunately, cases of fatal air embolization have been reported secondary to gas insufflation during arthroscopy in patients with intra-articular fractures.

Liquid Media

Irrigation with a liquid medium allows good visualization at constant pressure achieved through outflow control with adjustable pumps or other hydrostatic systems. Minor bleeding as well as debris can be washed out with this method alone. It has been found important that inflow should go through the sheath of the optical system to allow continuously good visualization. If suction-shaver systems are used, additional inflow cannulas are necessary in other parts of the knee joint, as these systems have higher fluid requirements which cannot be satisfied through the sheath alone.

The relationship beteen intra-articular pressure and pump capacity, measured by pressure and flowrate, follows simple hydrodynamic principles and has been known for some time. This must take into account the capacity of the pump, the modulus of elasticity of the human knee joint (as yet unknown), and the flow rate to the outside and into the surrounding tissues. These theoretical considerations have led to the conclusions discussed below.

Different methods for bringing the selected liquid medium into the joint through infusion tubing and cannulae are available:

1. gravity,
2. RPM-controlled pump,
3. Pressure– and flow rate–controlled pump.

Gravity. Adequate intra-articular pressure can be achieved by elevating a fluid container above the level of the knee. Advantages of this method are its simplicity and the fact that it does not require additional devices. A disadvantage is that large-bore cannulae are necessary and that pressure build-up is slow and the flow rate is low (Fig. **17**).

RPM-controlled pump. The pump with preset RPM is a useful instrument for the experienced surgeon. However, if the surgeon is distracted, the pump will continue to operate at the preset rate and can produce excessive intra-articular pressure. In addition, continuous intraoperative adjustment is necessary, either by the surgeon or by an assistant.

Pressure– and flow rate–controlled pump. A pump which allows control of intra-articular pressure and flow rate is the most desirable device. The maximal pressure is preset by the surgeon depending on the proposed procedure and the individual anatomy of the patient's knee joint; the flow rate can be individualized depending on the requirements during the operation. If the knee is tight or a high flow rate is necessary (for example, in the case of large amounts of debris), pressure and flow rate can be adjusted as needed.

An experienced and skillful surgeon may be able to obtain equally satisfactory results with an RPM-controlled pump. Excessive intra-

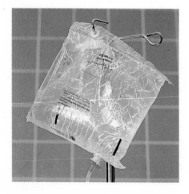

Fig. **17**   Gravity irrigation system. The simplest and safest irrigation system is a bag with irrigation fluid. If the bag is hung appropriately high above the surgical field, distention of the joint is sufficient for diagnostic arthroscopy. If glass bottles are used, a vent that serves as a bacterial filter has to be used. Because of their small capacity, they have to be changed frequently

articular pressure or cessation of flow with subsequent poor visibility cannot always be avoided, however. We feel that pressure-controlled pumps are preferable in order to make sure that excessive pressure peaks do not occur (Figs. **18** and **19**).

Attempts at controlling the pressure with a safety valve in the outflow tract have failed due to difficulties with sterilization and calibration.

Typical pressure curves obtained with different systems are shown in Fig. **20**. Constant filling status of the joint without excessive intra-articular pressure and rapid orientation in the joint are best achieved with the use of pressure– and flow rate–controlled pumps.

When arthroscopy is done with a liquid medium, special attention has to be paid to the outflow cannula, because it regulates flow rate and intra-articular pressure. Depending on its shape and caliber, the cannula may become clogged with debris. The blockage can be eliminated by introducing a mandrin into the cannula or by removing the obstruction under direct vision.

Any colorless isotonic solution can be used as distention and irrigation fluid in arthroscopy. Inexpensive electrolyte solutions are very useful, except in intra-articular electrosurgery where electrolyte-free solutions must be used. These are the same solutions that are used for electro-resection in urologic surgery (Table **4**).

Although extravasation of fluid through tears in the synovium and the capsule have been noticed, the risks of fluid irrigation during arthros-

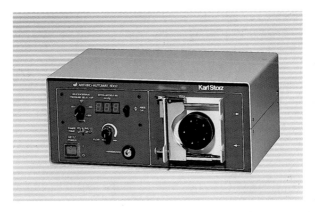

Fig. **18**   For arthroscopic purposes, a special pump is available with individually adjustable maximum and minimum pressures and flow rate. With an applied tourniquet, a pressure limitation of 180–200 mmHg has proved to be appropriate

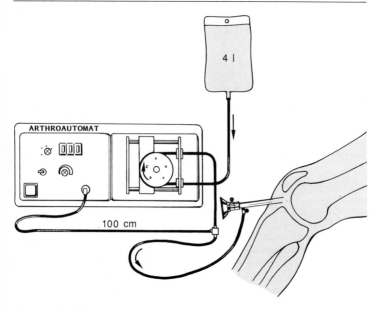

Fig. **19** Schematic drawing of the connection of an arthroscopy pump. An integrated pressure transducer with a filter for bacteria is connected to the system with T-tubing

Table **4**   Characteristics of liquid media

	pH	Osmolality	Conductivity
Isotonic solutions	5.7	Isoosmolar	Conducting
Water	7.0	Hypoosmolar	Conducting
Synovium	7.0–7.3	300 mosmol	Conducting
Sorbitol-mannitol solution	4.3–4.7	178 mosmol	Nonconducting

copy are not high, as absorption of the fluid is usually rapid. In several thousand arthroscopies, no serious side effects were noted.
The controversy over the use of a gas or a liquid medium for joint distention in arthroscopy has now been resolved. Gas is used exclusively for diagnostic arthroscopy, while liquid media are chosen for surgical applications.

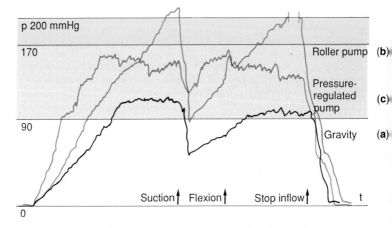

Fig. 20   Pressure within the knee joint during gravity irrigation (**a**, black line), during irrigation using a pump with controlled speed (**b**, blue line), and using a pump with controlled pressure and flow rate (**c**, red line). Advantages of the latter device: the slower pressure-decrease, the rapid pressure-increase in the low-pressure zone crease, the rapid pressure-increase in the low-pressure zone with slower pressure-increase as the filling process reaches its peak, and the avoidance of pressure peaks

Choice of Approach

Several portals have been employed for insertion of the arthroscope. The anterior approaches are widely used (that is, the scope is introduced through the capsule via a lateral or medial parapatellar route at the level of the inferior pole of the patella or the joint line). These approaches allow adequate examination of the knee joint. For special indications, a midpatellar lateral or a suprapatellar approach may be indicated. The latter route permits good visualization of the patella.

The central approach (Fig. **46** ff) provides a good overview of the joint space after perforation of the patellar tendon. The tendon supports the arthroscope and facilitates its manipulation inside the joint. Other advantages of this approach are a maximal field of vision inside the knee, the fact that it allows rapid orientation with the tibial plateau as a guide, and that it is easy to learn. The principle of this approach is the central access to the knee joint, not the central perforation of the patellar tendon. If the tibial tubercle is located laterally, access may occasionally be made from the medial side of the tendon.

The possible disadvantage of perforating the patellar tendon may be neglected if arthroscopy is done under general anesthesia. Delayed onset of pain is very rare. The tendon must be perforated with a quick stab of the trocar and not with drilling motions to avoid damage to a larger area of the tendon.

Since the arthroscope is easily moved between the cruciate ligaments and the femoral condyles, the central approach allows relatively easy visualization of the medial and lateral parts of the posterior compartment of the knee. The areas that cannot be visualized are much smaller than they are with other anterior approaches, which allow a good view of the posterior compartment only if the cruciate ligaments are incompetent. Even a minor mistake in the selection of the access site can make visualization of the ipsilateral part of the posterior joint compartment extremely difficult. With a 30°, scope, the central approach permits complete inspection of the medial and lateral capsule, the posterior oblique ligament and the two collateral ligaments, provided the capsule can be stretched sufficiently.

With the anteromedial or the anterolateral approaches, the femoral condyle, a synovial plica or Hoffa's fat pad can impede inspection of the contralateral part of the joint; the central approach does not present this problem.

The posterior part of the lateral capsule, which is located behind the femoral insertion of the popliteal muscle, cannot be visualized with any of the anterior approaches. It can only be inspected from a posterolateral approach with exact determination of the portal to avoid damage to articular cartilage and menisci. The same is true for the posteromedial part of the capsule.

It is important to choose the correct approach for the diagnostic or therapeutic problem at hand. If a lesion of the medial capsule is suspected, a central or a medial approach should be chosen, which allows optimal visualization even of the posterior oblique system. The central or the posterolateral approaches are best suited for examination of the lateral compartment. For inspection of the patellofemoral region, the suprapatellar approach is useful, even though this part of the joint can be examined from any of the anterior approaches as well. The central approach is best suited for evaluation of the gliding path of the patella and possible lateralization.

Fig. **21**   Blind spots. From the different approaches to the knee, only certain ▶ parts of the joint space can be visualized because of the multiple anatomical compartments and the column construction of the condyles. There are considerable differences between the various approaches. The largest visible surface and all important structures can be visualized through the central approach

Fig. **21**

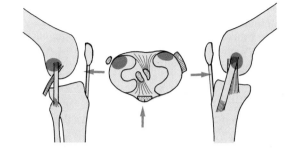

a Blind spots
from the central
approach

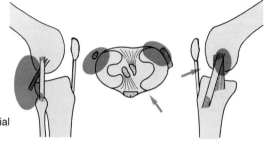

b Blind spots
from the anteromedial
approach

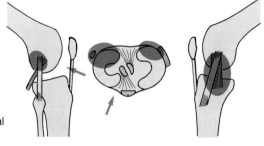

c Blind spots
from the anterolateral
approach

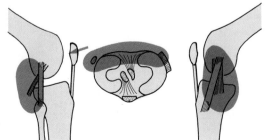

d Blind spots
from the midpatellar
approach

The central approach allows easy and safe access into the joint with an optimal field of vision, even into the posterior aspects of the knee joint. We believe that it is the most suitable approach for diagnostic and therapeutic arthroscopy, and that the other routes should be reserved for special indications (Fig. **21**).

Selection of Instruments

Optical systems, video recording, and video documentation

Telescopes with the universally accepted angulation (25−30° for regular scopes and 70° for special indications), in combination with the option to advance the tip of the scope into more distant areas of the joint, allow inspection of almost all intra-articular structures (Figs. **22−24**). The 30° scope does not require special training; use of the 70° scope requires training and adaptation since the field of vision is directed laterally. The straight or zero scope does not offer any advantages. More recently, special wide-angle scopes with a 110° field of vision have been developed; these scopes are preferable to the 85−90° angulations used in the past. They have the advantage that peripherally located loose bodies or other structures can occasionally be visualized.

While diagnostic arthroscopy can be performed without video equipment, sterile technique demands its use in arthroscopic surgery. With a

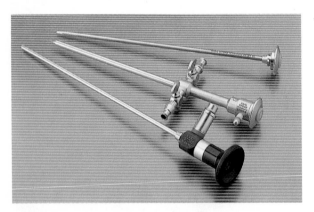

Fig. **22** The arthroscope in common used consists of a lens (bottom) with laterally attached light cable. A sheath with a sharp and a blunt trocar is used to introduce the instrument into the joint to protect the optical system from bending and breaking. The sheath also contains the irrigation port for gas or liquids

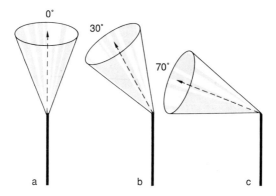

Fig. **23**   The arthroscopes of most manufactures allow a significant extension of the field of vision when the instrument is rotated and a 30° or even 70° lens is used. In most cases, the 30° lens is sufficient and only for special applications should it be exchanged for the 70° lens

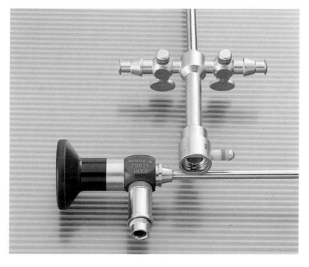

Fig. **24**   Details of the arthroscope. The vertical entrance of light into the optical system (below) and the valve system, with inflow for the distention medium are clearly visible

small chip camera it is possible to operate under completely sterile conditions, and the surgeon can work standing upright.

In addition, the entire operation can be recorded on magnetic tape for documentation and teaching purposes. We believe that this technology will advance to a point where printouts on paper will be possible which can be given directly to the referring physician and inserted into the patient's chart.

Hand instruments

A variety of instruments is required for diagnostic and surgical arthroscopy. Every surgeon should choose his or her own instruments from the large selection that is offered by the equipment companies (Figs. **25–31**).

A probing hook is a basic necessity. The hook should be calibrated for size and tip length and can serve as a gauge for the size of structures inside the joint. This is supplemented by a variety of other instruments. We prefer instruments with straight stems and differently shaped tips to the curved devices offered by some equipment companies. All instruments should have their predetermined breaking points located outside

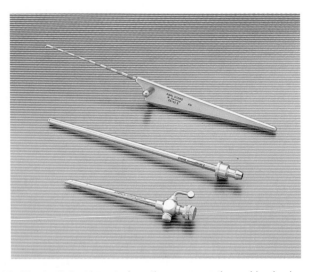

Fig. **25** The basic instruments for arthroscopy are the probing hook and the suction device. Furthermore, an outflow cannula, preferably with controlled flow, is necessary (should be disposable)

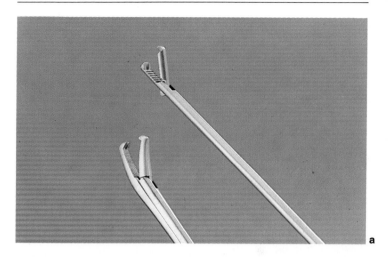

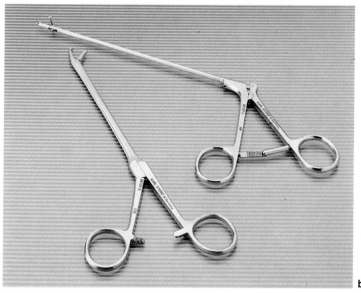

Fig. **26** Instruments to grasp an intra-articular body are equipped with teeth or small grooves on their branches. They can be locked temporarily to allow the surgeon to free his or her hand without losing tissue contact

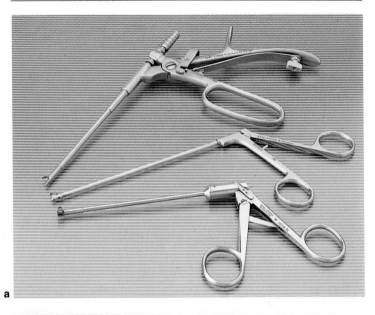

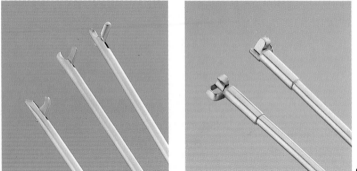

Fig. 27   Hand instruments to cut and resect intra-articular structures. These basket forceps remove small pieces of tissue and transport them into the joint space. After their use, suctioning of the joint is mandatory

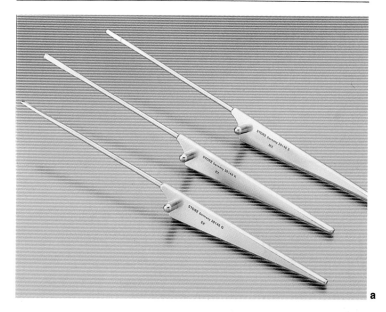

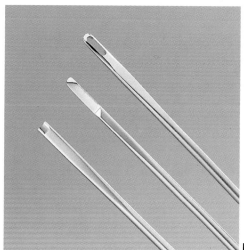

Fig. **28** Knifes and curettes for arthroscopy allow directed and exact cutting and removal of tissue

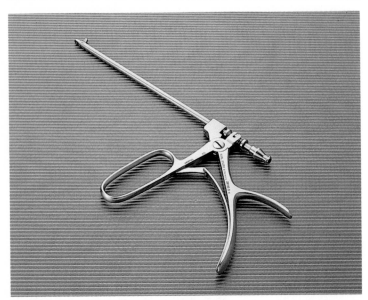

Fig. **29** The basket forceps with incorporated suction system allows one to suction free-floating particles between the branches of the forceps and then to remove them from the joint

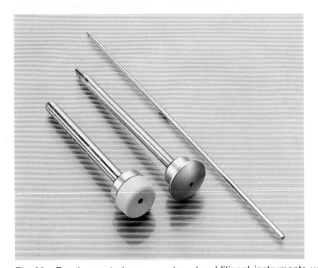

Fig. **30** For the posterior compartment, additional instruments were developed that are brought in through a separate portal which is defined using a needle under arthroscopic control

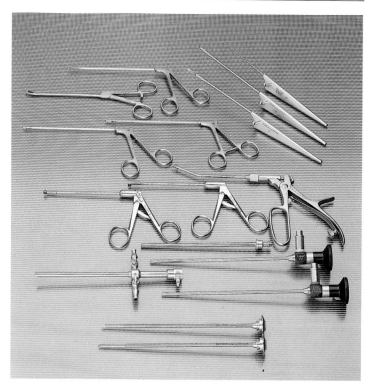

Fig. **31** The set depicted here has served well as a basic instrument set in several thousand diagnostic and surgical arthroscopies

the joint and movements of the different devices should be minimal inside the joint. Direct comparison between the different instruments will allow the surgeon the make his or her choice.

Table **5** lists the basic instruments as well as the drapes and dressings we like to use.

Power Systems

For synovectomy and chondroplasty, several power instruments have been developed which allow not only removal of these tissues in small particles but also their evacuation from the joint using (moderate)

Table 5   Basic arthroscopy set

1. Instruments (sterile)	2. Optical system (sterile)
a) Probing hook	a) 30° scope
b) Large grasping forceps	b) 70° scope
c) Small grasping forceps	c) Light cable
d) Hooked scissors	d) Camera
e) Basket forceps (straight)	e) Sheath
f) Basket forceps (upward bent broad)	f) Sharp trocar
	g) Blunt trocar
g) Basket forceps (90° angled, right)	
h) Basket forceps (90° angled, left)	
i) Rosette knife	
j) Smillie knife	
k) Suction device	
l) Skin forceps	
m) Needle holder	
n) Suture scissors	
o) Towel clips	
3. Additional Equipment (not sterile)	4. Additional Equipment (sterile)
a) Tourniquet	a) Extremity drape
b) U-drape	b) Stocking
c) Leg holder	c) Y-drape
d) Special knee cushion (Fig. 43)	d) Water tubing
e) Polster	e) Outflow cannula
f) Water bag (for irrigation)	f) Drape for camera
g) Pelvic support	g) Sponges, padding, bandages

negative hydrostatic pressure. A high flow rate is absolutely essential to ensure a constant suction effect. With these electrically or compressed-air driven systems, it is possible to remove abnormal free-floating or fixed bodies from the joint. Several reports in the literature indicate good results, but it must be pointed out that these instruments can be dangerous for healthy parts of the joint.

The choice between electrically driven instruments and devices powered by compressed air must be made by the surgeon according to local availability. Disposable equipment is on the market as well as instruments that can be sterilized (Figs. **32, 33**).

This technology has made significant advances. Instruments with forward and reverse gears are available and oscillating tools with controlled speed for different types of tissues. Equipment for tissue resection and for arthroplasty can also be obtained (Figs. **34, 90, 91**).

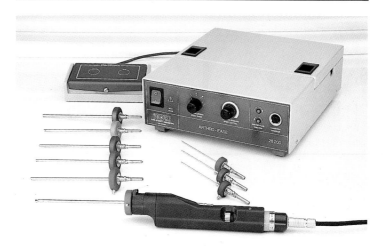

Fig. **32**   Motorized system for intra-articular cutting

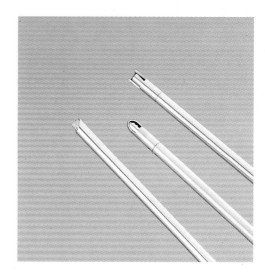

Fig. **33**   Working tips
for different shavers
are either side-cutting
or end-cutting. Their
effect is enhanced by
moderate suction

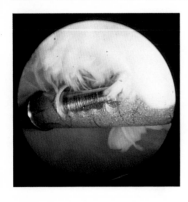

Fig. **34**   The shaver within the joint during the resection of cartilage (technique see Fig. **90**).

Electroresection

Electroresection is widely used now, especially for meniscus tissue. For these procedures, a liquid medium is required like that used for transurethral resection in urological surgery. We use sorbitol-mannitol solutions routinely during arthroscopy; this allows us to use electroresection whenever we think it is indicated. With a unipolar resection knife which is shaped like a probing hook, the structures can be placed under tension and then cut with preset pressure or tension. For high-frequency surgery of the meniscus, the same rules apply as they do for coagulation during open surgery. Correct positioning of the neutral electrode must checked before the procedure is started.

The combination of probing hook and electroresection knife is very effective (Fig. **35**). The dual use makes frequent changes of instruments unnecessary. It must be said, however, that these instruments are not yet optimally developed. The transition area between conductive and insulated material is still inadequate, as are the bending properties under tension.

Electroresection is limited to simple cutting procedures; the structures to be cut must be placed under tension, and a third incision into the joint is necessary in order to pass a forceps which holds the tissue (Fig. **36**).

The zone of tissue necrosis after electroresection is only a few micrometers thick (Fig. **37**), and permanent damage is not expected.

Electroresection obviously does not affect the meniscus alone (Figs. **38, 39**). Other tissues can be damaged if the technique is used in an uncontrolled manner. As the intra-articular space is relatively narrow, touching of other tissues cannot always be avoided during the procedure. It is not known whether cartilage lesions heal after electrical injury.

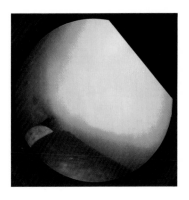

Fig. 35   The electroresection knife shaped like a probing hook, pointed at the lateral retinaculum

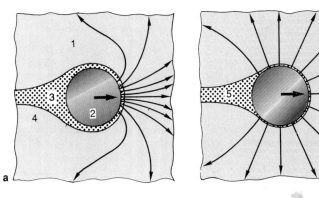

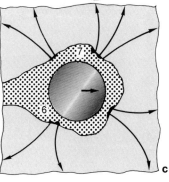

Fig. 36   Procedures for the electroresection of the meniscus. **a** Cutting at optimal power. **b** Cutting with insufficient power, initial cutting phase. **c** Cutting with too much power, excess energy. 1) tissue, 2) wire loop, 3) vapor, 4) high ohm tissue surface, 5) cutting channel 6) light arc, 7) deep necroses

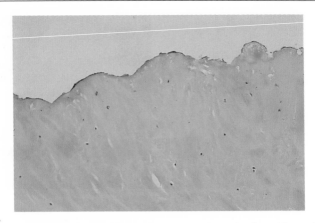

Fig. **37**   The necrotic zone of the removed meniscus is about 50 μm thick. Serious damage to the joint is not to be expected from these degradation products

Electroresection allows immediate coagulation of bleeders which makes its use for lateral retinacular release preferable to other surgical techniques. Before the procedure is terminated, the tourniquet should be released and the joint surfaces inspected. With properly adjusted pressure, the bleeding points can be visualized and coagulated. *A gas medium is contraindicated for this procedure.*

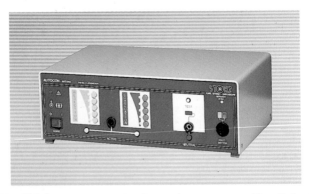

Fig. **38**   High-frequency apparatus for meniscus surgery, with optimized cutting power according to Fig. **39 b**

Opponents of electroresection emphasize that they can achieve the same effect with simple hand instruments which do not endanger healthy parts of the joint. Supporters of the method point out that they can achieve a rapid and optimal effect by simple introduction of the hook-shaped resection knife. Newer technologies are being developed for resection procedures inside the joint, for example, laser energy to cut tissue. Their place in arthroscopic surgery is undetermined at the present time.

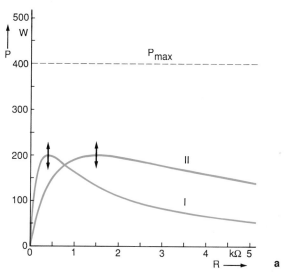

Fig. **39** Power output of high-frequency generators.
a Conventional high-frequency generators (output adjusted by hand). The power output (P) depends on the electric resistance (R) of the patient at any particular moment. Every high-frequency generator supplies a maximum output at a certain resistance; the power decreases if the resistance is higher or lower. As a rule, high-frequency generators are constructed to achieve maximum output approximately at the most likely resistance value of the patient. Curve I was measured at a generator for urology. In these operations, the patient resistance is mostly in a range between 400 Ω and 1.5 kΩ. Curve II was obtained with a generator for arthroscopic operations where the most frequent patient resistance values are between 1.5 and 4 kΩ. The curves can be adjusted manually toward higher or lower output, as shown schematically by the arrows. However, once an adjustment has been set, only those values can be attained that lie on the relevant curve. The maximum possible performance (Pmax) is limited to 400 W to comply with official safety rules

Fig. 39 b on page 46

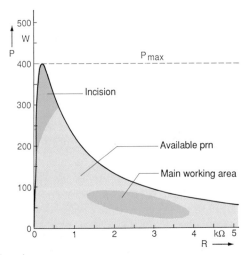

Fig. **39** continued
b High-frequency generators with automatic power regulation (light-arc controlled regulation). Some high-frequency generators are on the market that
automatically adjust their performance to the actual power requirement. This
automatic control is effected by electronically measuring the sparking distance
of the small electric arc between the probing hook and the tissue and automatically adjusting it to the smallest possible value. Such a generator can make all
outputs available at any patient-resistance value if they are below an output-
limit curve, as shown by the blue areas. As the first incision is made, patient
resistance (R) is relatively low, and high outputs are delivered with rapid initial
incision ("incision"). Once the incision is under way, patient resistance (R) rises
rapidly to a high level, and the output required is very low. At this stage, the
generator adjusts the output to a level far below the limit curve. On an average,
the output passed to the patient is considerably lower than with manually
adjusted generators ("main working area"). Advantages resulting from this are:
fewer and less extensive necroses, uniform quality of incision, fewer air and
gas bubbles, less hazard for the patient, and greatly reduced disturbances for
video systems

Arthroscopic Work Place

There is a variety of technical possibilities available for the variety of possible diagnoses and therapeutic procedures. Every surgeon will rapidly develop his or her own method and select the preferred instruments for it. All methods have the use of a light source, increased pressure, an optical system, and video technology in common. This equipment is combined with other devices to form the arthroscopist's work place.

This work place should be easy to operate, should allow rapid orientation, should provide sterile conditions, and should be easily accessible for the surgeon. We have developed our own compact version of an arthroscopic work place which can be placed on a special cart or stand.

This unit permits the surgeon to work either sitting or standing, looking straight ahead, and with an optimal position of the hands (provided a video system is used).

With this type of work place, the surgeon can perform arthroscopic operations under ergonomic conditions where the instruments are easily moved into the proper positions, are not exposed to being jostled, and are easy to store (Fig. **40**).

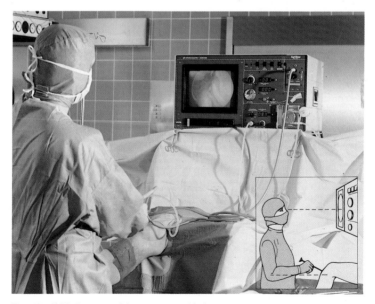

Fig. **40** With integrated instruments, "Arthrocompact" features easy operation, easy sterilization, and ergonomic working conditions. The TV screen for viewing can be adjusted to the working position of the surgeon

The Arthroscopic Operation

Informed Consent

Arthroscopy of the knee, like all other invasive procedures, involves the risks of infection, damage to nerves and blood vessels and thromboembolic complications. Besides these general complications, specific problems such as gas emphysema and compartment syndromes must be mentioned to the patient.

In addition, the consequences of the arthroscopic procedure have to be discussed:

— A patient with a fresh posttraumatic hemarthrosis must be advised that repair or reconstruction of ligaments, (partial) resection or reattachment of a meniscus may have to be performed during the same anesthesia.
— If arthroscopic surgery is planned, the patient should be told that arthrotomy may be required, should endoscopic maneuvers fail or an instrument break in the joint.
— In cases of acute arthroscopy, the patient should be informed that subsequent definitive repair may be necessary.

Educational pamphlets containing basic information about the technique and the practical aspects of arthroscopy are helpful.

The rehabilitation program should be discussed, as well as possible findings during arthroscopy and treatment of possible complications (for example, infection or effusion).

Preparation and Positioning

Preparations for arthroscopy are not different from those for any other joint operation. For elective procedures, preparation includes preoperative disinfection without shaving of the knee and a shower or bath on the day before surgery. The anesthesiologist will also make his or her necessary preoperative arrangements.

In the operating room, the patient is positioned on an operating table which should have an adjustable leg part if arthroscopy is to be done on the hanging leg (Fig. **41**). Other authors prefer a normal position and adjust the patient's knee during the operation. It is advisable to support the leg so that it hangs freely with the knee in flexion once the leg support of the table is lowered. A U-shaped thigh holder is helpful for applying varus and valgus stress to the knee during the procedure (Fig. **42**). We do not recommend a rigid leg holder, especially with an integrated tourniquet. Iatrogenic lesions caused by faulty positioning, such as compression of the peroneal nerve, must be avoided.

Positioning the patient with hanging legs produces hyperlordosis of the lumbar spine which may result in lower back pain after the operation.

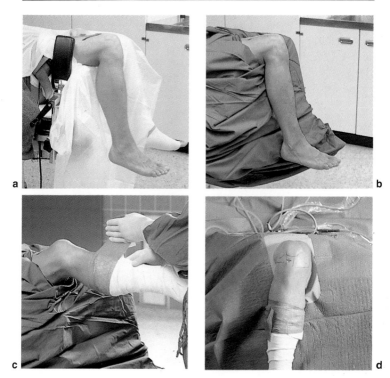

Fig. 41   Preparation for arthroscopy: **a** The thigh is positioned in the leg holder so that varus and valgus stress can be applied. The lower limb hangs down and can be flexed to 120°. The tourniquet is positioned proximal to the leg holder; it is well padded and covered with Vi-drape. **b** After disinfection, the first drape is applied in the anteroom; this is followed by a second spray disinfection. **c** The lower leg is wrapped in a waterproot stocking and is separated from the surgical field with a Vi-drape. **d** Second sterile draping with a disposable drape with a central hole. The camera is covered with sterile tubing and placed on the field

We remedy this by placing a sterilized pillow under the contralateral leg; the pillow is fastened with a strap placed under the patient's back to prevent its displacement during the operation (Fig. **43**).

To avoid operating on the wrong leg, the affected knee is marked with an indelible felt pen while the patient is still awake (Fig. **44**).

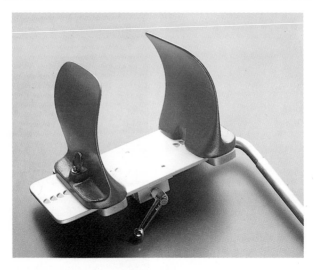

Fig. **42**   The leg holder facilitates opening of the lateral and medial knee compartments with varus or valgus stress

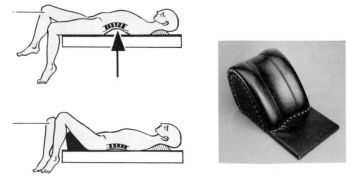

Fig. **43**   With hanging legs, hyperlordosis of the lumbar spine can occur, which results in postoperative pain. This is prevented almost completely by the use of a special pillow placed under the leg not being operated on

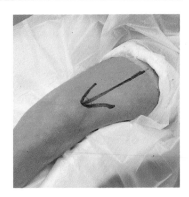

Fig. **44**   The leg to be operated on is marked with a water-resistant marker to avoid confusion between right and left while the patient is asleep

Maintenance and Sterilization of Instruments

Since the equipment used is very expensive, it should undergo careful and regular maintenance.

Lenses and fiber optics are particularly susceptible to damage. The lens can be damaged by autoclaving. Bending of the optical system can result in the breakage of fibers. This damage can be repaired, however. The light guides contain many fine fiber bundles which are surrounded by protective materials. If the light cable is bent, single fibers can break which will eventually result in destruction of the optical system. Bending of the cable through a diameter of less than 20 cm should be avoided.

Video cameras have become more robust but they, too, have to be protected against inadvertent autoclaving. The manufacturers recommend disinfection with glutaraldehyde. We usually place the camera in sterile plastic tubing which can be done without difficulty.

All hand and power instruments have to be cleaned between and after cases and should be treated with a silicone oil. Rasps, shavers, etc. must be cared for according to the manufacturer's maintenance instructions.

Because the instruments can fall during the procedure, as with any other device, back-up instruments must be available, especially a second 30° scope, a light cable, and a replacement bulb for the light source.

Completing the Arthroscopic Procedure

Diagnostic arthroscopy is usually completed after irrigation of the joint, an occasional biopsy, removal of all instruments, skin closure and application of the dressing. Since the incision is small, a separate closure of the capsule is not necessary. A good cosmetic result can be achieved even without formal skin closure. A compression dressing should be applied prophylactically in the operating room.

After an arthroscopic operation with wound closure and surgical dressing, immobilizion of the joint or rapid mobilization (for example with a motorized splint) will have to be considered. Fixation with a plaster splint for two days may be justified in some cases. For most patients, however, rapid mobilization without weight-bearing according to general orthopedic principles is preferable.

There will always be procedures with an undesired outcome. Occasionally, the operation will have to be terminated prematurely as a result of technical difficulties. If fragments of the meniscus remain in the joint, the patient must be informed that the procedure may be repeated when swelling has subsided (usually after approximately four weeks). A broken instrument should be removed immediately, if necessary by arthrotomy.

Arthrotomy During the Same Anesthesia

If a cruciate ligament rupture or a longitudinal tear of a meniscus is diagnosed during acute arthroscopy, definitive surgical repair should be performed during the same anesthesia after renewed disinfection and draping of the operative field.

We would like to caution against doing arthrotomy several days after arthroscopy; there are indications that the risk of infection is then much higher than it is with either operation performed alone or with both procedures done in the same sitting.

Before a delayed secondary procedure is performed, the skin must be in good condition, there should be no crusts or purulent coating in the area to be operated on.

The length of the arthroscopic procedure has a definite influence on duration and intensity of postoperative discomfort; prolonged perfusion of the joint causes the tissues to swell which may change the anatomical relationships.

Although the low incidence of infection following arthroscopy does not allow statistical conclusions, we must assume that the risk of infection increases with increasing duration of the procedure.

An average arthroscopic operation (with the exclusion of ligament repair, synovectomy or abrasion chondroplasty) should not take longer than 60 minutes. After that time, the procedure should be converted to an arthrotomy.

If a meniscus fragment or a loose body is lost in the joint during arthroscopic surgery, a careful and systematic search with the arthroscope should be made for it first before arthrotomy is performed.

Orientation within the joint is usually better with an arthroscope than with a small or medium arthrotomy. Even pieces of broken instruments can often be removed using the arthroscope and a suitable grasping forceps.

Suspicion of Infection

Infection of a joint can be an indication for arthroscopy, or the diagnosis can be made during arthroscopy for other indications.

For a known joint empyema, arthroscopy is an excellent method for decompressing the joint and evacuating the damaging infectious products; it can also be used to establish continuous irrigation, which should be left in place until negative cultures have been obtained on three consecutive days.

Occasionally one is surprised to find a productive synovitis which justifies the suspicion of a joint infection.

In these cases we recommend biopsy, and culture, followed by immediate irrigation with simple irrigation fluid and later with antibiotic solutions.

We prefer an irrigation fluid consisting of Ringer's solution with a combination of neomycin sulfate, bacitracin and polymyxin b to irrigate the knee for 30−40 minutes with an intra-articular pressure of 60 mmHg (corresponds to an elevation of 1 m above the knee for hydrostatic irrigation).

Problems and Complications

Incidence

Arthroscopy has been found to be a procedure with very few complications. Transient effusions (usually hemarthroses) are seen in approximately 10% of all cases while other, mostly minor, complications occur in less than 1%. However, there may be an unidentified number of complications which are not immediately apparent and can only be suspected. Unexplained long-lasting effusions or postoperative pain should encourage the surgeon to re-evaluate the procedure for possible errors in technique.

Infection

In large international studies, the risk of infection after arthroscopy was found to be minimal. The reasons for this may be found in a well-functioning team; the constant irrigation of the joint with liquid media may be an important prophylactic factor. It is a well-known fact that the occurrence of an infection is not only determined by organism and mode of inoculation but also by the number of pathogens.

Fluid Leak

Injuries to the synovial membrane and the joint capsule can result in leakage of fluid into the surrounding tissues where it is usually resorbed without sequelae within 30−60 minutes. Diuretics are not necessary. We have not observed any so-called overinfusions of saline solution. The only compartment syndromes of the leg described in the literature were observed following acute arthroscopy in patients with injury to the head of the fibula.

Gas Leak

Leakage of gas into the surrounding tissues has been looked upon as an annoying but not serious complication. Recently, however, two fatal cases of gas embolism have been reported during arthroscopy in patients with intra-articular fractures. We feel that gas should be used with great caution for joint distention and never for patients with fresh fractures.

Damage to Articular Cartilage

It can be assumed that any instrument touching the articular cartilage causes some damage to it. Wrongly selected instruments, abrupt movements of the instruments deep inside the joint, or electroresection can cause damage to other tissues; this should be avoided as much as possible. Removal of larger areas of cartilage probably leaves permanent damage, but minor injuries eventually heal without sequelae.

The risks of difficult arthroscopic procedures are discussed in the description of these procedures.

General Risks

Deep venous thrombosis of the calf has been seen infrequently, like it has been after other surgical procedures.

The tourniquet represents an inherent risk, and the surgeon must pay attention to proper placement and appropriate pressure. The risk of operating on the wrong knee can be avoided by identifying the correct knee with an indelible felt marker before the operation while the patient is still awake (Fig. **44**).

Breakage of instruments inside the joint was a problem during the introductory years of arthroscopy. This problem has been corrected in the meantime. The newer instruments have predetermined breaking points which are located outside the actual joint space.

Indications, Contraindications and Alternative Methods

Indications

Like with all other operations, the indications for arthroscopy can be divided into absolute and relative indications.

Absolute indications are those conditions for which arthrotomy was previously necessary but which can now be treated arthroscopically.

Relative indications should be discussed between the patient and the physician, and possible risks should be weighed against the diagnostic value or the expected improvement in the patient's condition, or both.

Diagnostic arthroscopy (Table **6**) is indicated for all clinical conditions in which the diagnosis cannot be clarified by examination alone. Arthroscopy may be useful if symptoms are present for which cause or location are not clear enough to establish a reasonable therapeutic approach. If the diagnosis is obvious, and age and location of the lesion can be determined, the extent of the damage may have to be clarified by arthroscopy to allow better therapeutic planning and to justify the proposed treatment. Arthroscopy can be useful in determining the nature of the pathology in forensic cases and for disability evaluation after injuries. However, since arthroscopy is a surgical procedure, its

Table **6**   Indications for diagnostic arthroscopy grouped by structures

1. Meniscus tear
    a) Diagnostic uncertainty
    b) Uncertainty about the exact location of the tear
    c) Associated injuries

2. Ligament injuries
    a) With instability: rule out associated injury
    b) Suspicion of acute ligament injury without instability (= hemarthrosis): absolute indication for arthroscopy
    c) Chronic instability (to plan surgery or rule out associated injuries)

3. Pathology of femur and patella
    a) Associated injuries (displaced fragments)
    b) Stages of arthrosis
    c) Evaluation of joint blockage of uncertain etiology

4. Synovial pathology
    a) Synovitis and effusion of unclear etiology
    b) Uncertain diagnosis, biopsy of synovial membrane
    c) Treatment planning

5. Follow-up of treatment results

use to clarify insurance questions should be limited to absolutely necessary indications.

Arthroscopy can be a valuable tool in some cases of known underlying disease or known trauma, such as capsular or ligamentous injury or osteochondritis dissecans. It can help us to determine whether treatment should be conservative or operative (arthroscopic surgery or arthrotomy). For example, diagnostic arthroscopy can be helpful in deciding whether a hemarthrosis with collateral ligament lesion can be treated by plaster immobilization (after exclusion of other internal joint lesions) or whether, in the case of osteochondritis dissecans, removal of a loose body or reattachment of the osteochondritic fragment via arthroscopy or via arthrotomy is required.

The transition from diagnostic to operative arthroscopy can be described as an "aggressive diagnostic procedure with conservative surgical treatment."

Only ten years ago, arthroscopy was felt to be indicated when clinical and radiological examination including arthrography could not provide an adequate explanation for the patient's symptoms. Because of the recent advances in technique, arthroscopic surgery is now used more often than diagnostic arthroscopy.

Some patients who have been under medical care for a long time will eventually require arthroscopic examination. The sequence of diagnostic steps to be followed is given in Table **7**. Adequate conservative treatment can occasionally establish the diagnosis by means of the therapeutic measures which seem to improve the condition and can help to avoid the arthroscopic procedure.

Once the decision to perform diagnostic arthroscopy has been made, the surgical team should be prepared to proceed with arthroscopic surgery if necessary.

While arthrotomy is always performed based on the patient's history and objective clinical findings, arthroscopic surgery often follows arthroscopic examination of an unclear knee problem.

In contrast to other authors, we have determined that arthroscopy should be performed only in cases with a clear indication for an

Table **7**   Step-by-step evaluation of diseases of the knee-joint leading up to arthroscopy

1. History
2. Clinical examination
3. X-rays
4. Empirical treatment
5. Arthroscopy

operation and not as a diagnostic procedure to be followed by an operative intervention if indicated by the arthroscopic findings. If an operation is not indicated, the procedure is carried out as a diagnostic arthroscopy under operative conditions (anesthesia, irrigation with a liquid medium). We believe that this serves the patient better and accommodates the operating room schedule better.

The indications for arthroscopic surgery can be classified according to the different structures forming the knee joint (Table **8**).

Arthroscopic operations of the knee can be divided into the following categories:

— resecting procedures,
— plastic procedures,
— reconstructive procedures.

This implies that even major procedures can be performed arthroscopically, for example, the reattachment of a loose body in osteochondritis dissecans, the suture of a meniscus tear, or the implantation of an artificial cruciate ligament.

Arthroscopy can be of value even when no pathology is found.

Patients in whom no pathological changes were detected during initial diagnostic arthroscopy often report considerable improvement of their

Table **8**   Indications for surgical arthroscopy grouped by structure

1. Synovium
   a) Biopsy
   b) Synovectomy
   c) Lysis of adhesions
   d) Division of plica
   e) Lateral release

2. Synovial space
   a) Lavage
   b) Loose bodies

3. Intra-articular structures
   a) Meniscectomy
   b) Suture of the meniscus
   c) Suture of cruciate ligaments

4. Cartilage
   a) Shaving of the patella
   b) Refixation of an osteochondritis dissecans fragment
   c) Chondroplasty

5. Bone
   a) Removal of osteophyte
   b) Pridie drilling
   c) Fixation of fracture

symptoms on follow-up visits. There is no objective explanation for this phenomenon, but the patient is relieved and can be assured that no abnormalities were found.

In addition, lavage of the joint during arthroscopy, the postoperative recovery period, physical therapy, and rehabilitation all have psychological and physical effects on the patient's condition.

These findings have been confirmed by multiple reports in the literature.

Contraindications

Contraindications for arthroscopy are usually outside the orthopedic specialty. We must caution against arthroscopy in patients with a fracture of the head of the fibula because of the danger of a compartment syndrome. Furthermore, the use of gas as an inflation medium when fractures are present in the joint carries the risk of gas emboli.

Infection may result from the presence of skin lesions. The anesthesiologist must consider the risks of anesthesia for an elective surgical procedure and must discuss these with the patient.

The surgeon has to decide whether a clear indication is present for the arthroscopic procedure. Diagnostic arthroscopy should not replace the clinical examination.

Other circumstances like those illustrated in Figure **45,** can make arthroscopy difficult or even impossible. These anatomic variations may represent contraindications to arthroscopic procedures.

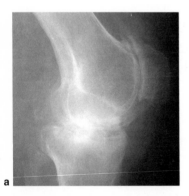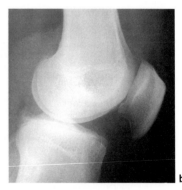

a   b

Fig. **45** Deformities and variations of the knee joint that make arthroscopy much more difficult are bony deformities with a reduced intra-articular space as it occurs in severe degenerative joint disease of the knee (**a**) or after traumatic or surgical changes. A patella baja (**b**) may also necessitate another approach if a central access route was planned

Technical incompetence, for example, the inability to deal with a trapped bucket handle tear, should be a contraindication to arthroscopic surgery.

Arthroscopy should be avoided if clinical examination dictates a different approach. A knee joint with a positive anterior drawer test but without symptoms of cartilage or synovial pathology is indicative of an isolated anterior cruciate ligament tear and should be treated with open surgical repair and should not be subjected to invasive diagnostic procedures such as arthroscopy.

Injuries which can be clearly diagnosed by radiological studies but cannot be handled by arthroscopic surgery should not be considered for diagnostic arthroscopy.

Alternative Methods

Before arthroscopy is used to clarify a pathological problem, one should evaluate whether other diagnostic methods could yield the same or better results. The objective must determine the choice of the procedure in all cases.

Arthrography as a supplement to routine radiographs has a much lower diagnostic accuracy than arthroscopy and does not allow immediate surgical treatment. It requires less equipment, however, and is less invasive.

Magnetic resonance imaging is expected to improve diagnostic evaluation of joint disorders in the future.

No other diagnostic procedure offers the advantage of immediate surgical treatment like arthroscopy does.

Arthrotomy enables the surgeon to perform most of the procedures that can be done arthroscopically. Both methods have their advantages and disadvantages. Further improvement of arthroscopic surgery can be expected in the future and may make alternative methods obsolete.

Diagnostic Arthroscopy

Principles and Indications

Diagnostic arthroscopy is used in patients with unclear findings or longstanding and therapy-resistant symptoms and before every arthroscopic operation. It is merely an examination of the joint surfaces; its ability to test function and tissue consistency is limited. Pain caused by biomechanical problems (for example, pain due to malalignment of the patella) is difficult to evaluate. Synovial biopsy should be done routinely and can provide valuable information about underlying diseases.

It is important to visualize the entire joint space, including posterior and lateral compartments since tears in the posteromedial compartment are frequently missed.

Experience has shown that even a "negative" arthroscopy can have a beneficial effect for a patient with a chronic painful knee condition (see "indications," Table **6**).

The diagnosis should be made in approximately 15 minutes (that is, all joint compartments must be evaluated within that time period including the appropriate function and probing tests).

One rule must be kept in mind during diagnostic arthroscopy: pain cannot be seen with the arthroscope.

Technique

Approach to the Joint

After appropriate preparation, the central approach is chosen because of its many advantages. The incision over the patellar tendon is transverse and follows the skin lines. It is usually in the medial portion of the patellar tendon (Fig. **46**). Medial and lateral joint line are determined by palpation, and the tendon is then perforated halfway between the joint line and the distal pole of the patella. The distance to the distal pole of the patella should be at least 0.5–1 cm. A slightly more medial approach should be chosen in case of a patella baja. The tendon should be punctured with a trocar using a quick stab and not with a drilling motion. The knee should be hanging in 90° of flexion, and the direction of the perforation should be parallel to the tibial plateau (Fig. **50a**).

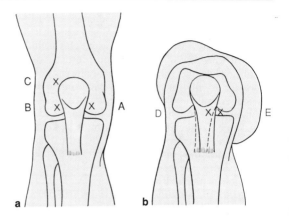

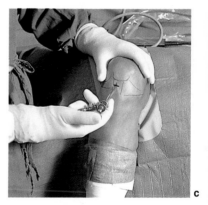

Fig. 46 Anterior standard approaches. The anteromedial and anterolateral approaches are widely used (A and B). The mid patella lateral approach allows good visualization of the patella (C). The central approach combines most of the advantages (D). Its position is – depending on the individual anatomy – in the medial third or directly medial of the patellar tendon (E). The photograph (c) shows the central approach after the landmarks are indicated using a sterile tissue pen

After perforation of the tendon, the sharp trocar is exchanged for a blunt obturator. This instrument is advanced until hard or soft resistance is met in the intercondylar notch (bone or cruciate ligament).

The scope is then advanced medially or laterally into the suprapatellar recess while the knee is gradually extended.

Care must be taken not to injure the articular cartilage of the trochlear groove and the undersurface of the patella (Fig. 50 b).

The blunt obturator is replaced by an arthroscope with a 30° lens, and the joint is inspected. Irrigation is then started and the joint space is distended rapidly, which allows good visualization of the suprapatellar recess.

As soon as the joint is sufficiently dilated, an outflow cannula is inserted under direct vision from a lateral suprapatellar portal, and a partially closed outflow valve is placed on it. This cannula should be inserted with the knee in 90° of flexion to prevent its impingement under the patella during the subsequent procedure. With this method, it is not necessary to fill the joint by puncturing it before the procedure is started. Probing hooks and surgical instruments can be inserted into the joint space through additional incisions on both sides to examine menisci and articular cartilage. It must be kept in mind, however, that anatomical structures as well as the arthroscope itself may block the way for additional instruments. For example, the femoral condyles may prevent access to the posterior horn if a contralateral approach is used. The anterior parts of the meniscus can be examinded with a probing hook from the ipsilateral side but can seldom be reached with surgical instruments. This makes an additional incision necessary from a slightly higher portal on the conralateral side (Fig. **47**). The anterior incisions are assigned to the respective parts of the meniscus (Fig. **48**). A paracentral portal is located approximately 1 cm above the tibial plateau and approximately 1.5 cm from the scope. From this portal, the posterior horn can be reached with suitable instruments. The procedure is facilitated by the parallel position of arthroscope and instruments.

This portal must be placed slightly higher to compensate for the thickness of the meniscus base.

The middle part of the meniscus can usually be reached without difficulty through an ipsilateral approach and with instruments that are angled approximately 90°. This portal is located slightly lower than that of the central approach and 4 cm medial or lateral to the midline; if possible this approach should be used first.

Using the probing hook, both menisci can be examined from this approach, as well as both cruciate ligaments and the undersurface of the patella. Just above it (approximately 2 cm higher and closer to the

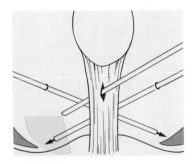

Fig. **47**   Central approach for the arthroscope through the patellar tendon. Additional medial and lateral incisions are used for insertion of the surgical instruments into the knee joint. Approach to the anterior compartment of the joint on the contralateral side: 2 cm to the side and 2 cm above the articulating surface on the contralateral side

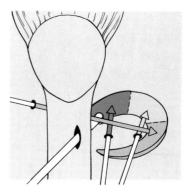

Fig. **48** Secondary anterior incisions depending on the location of the pathology findings

Central approach:	1 cm above the plateau	central
Paracentral approach:	1 cm above the plateau	1.5 cm to the side
Medial 1:	0.5 cm above the plateau	4 cm to the side
Medial 2:	2 cm above the plateau	3 cm to the side

midline) we find the best approach to the anterior horn of the opposite meniscus using angled instruments and to the middle section of that meniscus using straight instruments.

The posterior portals are more difficult to determine. Knowledge of the shape of the femoral condyles and of the anatomy of the ligaments is a prerequisite. The puncture site can be determined by a line approximately 1 cm above the tibial plateau which extends from the posterior edge of the medial collateral ligament to approximately 2 cm posterior to this point. The lateral puncture site is also located 1 cm above the level of the tibial plateau in the triangle between the femur, collateral ligament and biceps tendon (Fig. **49 a, b**).

The posterior curvature of the femoral condyles and the possible necessity to advance to the opposite side may compel one to use a posterior approach.

The relationship of this line to the knee joint is demonstrated in Figure **49 c.** To protect the neurovascular bundle in the popliteal space, the knee must be held in a flexed position.

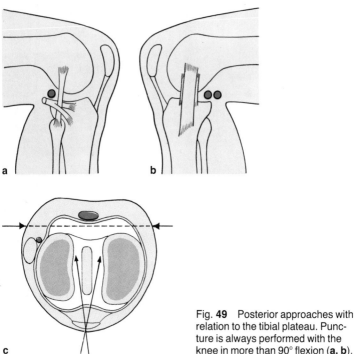

Fig. **49** Posterior approaches with relation to the tibial plateau. Puncture is always performed with the knee in more than 90° flexion (**a**, **b**).

Posteromedial 1:	1 cm above the plateau	behind the medial collateral ligament/posterior oblique ligament complex
Posteromedial 2:	1 cm above the plateau	2 cm behind the femoral condyles
Posterolateral:	1 cm above the plateau	between femoral condyle and biceps muscle

The posterior approaches are about 1 cm behind the posterior connecting line between the two femoral condyles (**c**). If the distance is too small, the instrument cannot be move sufficiently within the joint space (caution: only in flexion!)

Examining the Joint Space

The knee joint is a multiform cavity which should be inspected from one portal in a standardized fashion using different positions with a 30° and a 70° arthroscope.

Every arthroscopist should develop his or her own routine for examining the knee. In this section we attempt to outline our own principles, which should lead to a quick, complete and thus efficient examination. The surgeon should always keep in mind that every movement inside the joint is a trauma in itself, and that manipulations of the various instruments should be reduced to an absolute minimum.

The angled scopes are of significant help; a wide-angle 30° scope allows visualization of a large area, and a significant field of vision can be obtained by simply rotating the scope inside the sheath without turning the whole instrument.

We have found the following routine to be helpful in examining the knee joint arthoscopically and describe it without a specific pathological process in mind (Fig. **50**).

Usually we design our approach so that the area with the suspected pathology is examined last, and we then proceed immediately with arthroscopic surgery, if that is indicated.

1. Insertion of the arthroscope. With the knee in 90° of flexion, the sharp trocar and sheath are introduced into the joint space parallel to the tibial plateau.

2. The suprapatellar recess. The scope is introduced into the suprapatellar recess with the aid of sheath and blunt obturator. Initially, the tip of the scope is in contact with the synovial membrane. After irrigation is started, the joint space opens up rapidly; the scope is withdrawn slightly, and the expanded joint cavity allows thorough examination of the suprapatellar recess, provided it is illuminated adequately.

The suprapatellar recess is examined for loose bodies, changes in the appearance of the synovial membrane, as well as pathological plicae and adhesions.

3. The undersurface of the patella and the trochlear groove. A wide field of vision is obtained by turning the scope 360° in the suprapatellar recess. The scope is rotated downward and, looking at the synovial cover of the distal femur, it is pulled back to the proximal end of the articular cartilage of the knee. The normal position of the patella is just above this point. The scope is now turned 180° (the lens faces upward) and the undersurface of the patella is inspected. Depending on the status of the collateral ligaments and the intra-articular pressure, the proximal part of the patella can be visualized by turning the scope more medially or laterally.

As the scope is withdrawn further, the articular cartilage of the trochlear groove comes into view.

In different positions of flexion, the extent of the frequently existing lateralization of the patella and possible ulcerations of its articular cartilage can be visualized (seen best with the 70° scope). The knee is then extended and the joint examined for possible parapatellar plica

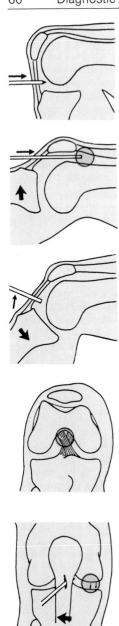

Fig. **50**   The route through the joint space.

a 1st step: The scope is introduced into the joint parallel to the tibial plateau with the knee in 90° of flexion

b 2nd step: Inspection of the superior recess during extension. The entire lining of the superior recess can be visualized by rotating, lateral motion and moving of the scope forward and backward

c 3nd step: During simultaneous flexion the scope is brought to the cartilage border, then rotated to inspect the undersurface of the patella; it is then advanced into the central compartment along the trochlear groove

d 4th step: The intercondylar space, with its boundaries and its contents, is examined by rotation and lateral motion of the scope

e 5th step: The medial compartment is opened under moderate valgus stress to visualize the main parts of the medial meniscus

f 6th step: By carefully rotating the scope —if necessary, with temporary extension of the knee—the circumference of the distal femur is visualized with the medial and lateral gutter. As an alternative, the scope can also be brought to the contralateral side over the anterior tibial plateau

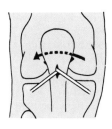

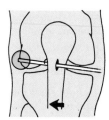

g 7th step: The lateral gutter and the popliteal recess can be inspected under valgus stress

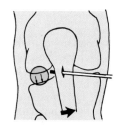

h 8th step: A change to varus stress allows inspection of the lateral joint compartment and the edge of the lateral meniscus

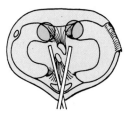

i 9th step: The scope is advanced into the posteromedial and posterolateral joint compartments; it is then rotated, or perhaps a change to the 70° system may be necessary

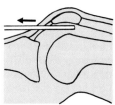

j 10th step: The scope is pulled back into the suprapatellar pouch, and the diagnostic procedure is completed with irrigation, suction and synovial biopsy

formation. Lateral and medial edges of the femur can be seen by rotating the scope appropriately. Besides injuries, for instance, a traumatic dislocation of the patella, a plica-shelf syndrome may be found in this area.

4. *The intercondylar notch.* The arthroscope is pulled back; the lens is turned downward toward the articular cartilage of the trochlear groove, and the knee is flexed 90°. The upper edge of the intercondylar notch can now be seen. When the scope is lowered slightly, one usually sees the so-called ligamentum mucosum, or in its absence, the anterior cruciate ligament. The anterior aspect of the intercondylar notch is visualized again by turning the scope. One should look for variations of the anterior cruciate ligament, the central edges of both femoral condyles (watch for osteochondritis dissecans) and possible bucket handle tears of the menisci.

5. *The medial joint space.* Pathological changes are most frequently found in this space. The scope is turned medially and slightly distally, and a mild valgus stress is applied to the knee. This allows good visualization of the anterior joint space. By gradually changing the position of flexion from 30° to 70°, the entire meniscus can generally be examined.

It is of particular importance to examine all visible parts of the meniscus with the probing hook to detect a possible hypermobility phenomenon. The undersurface occasionally shows degenerative tears which should also be demonstrated with the probing hook. To examine the opposite side, the scope is directed laterally following the bone–cartilage interface of the intercondylar notch, guiding it around the cruciate ligament and the ligamentum mucosum. Another possible route is through the suprapatellar recess. This, however, involves the risk of damage to the articular cartilage, especially for the beginner. It occurs most frequently when the arthroscope is advanced far into the joint, and movements of the instrument can then gouge out cartilage fragments.

6. *The periphery of the femoral condyle.* The cartilage edges of both femoral condyles can be demonstrated by passing the scope around the circumference of the joint and changing the compartment at the same time.

7. *The lateral joint space.* Lateral meniscus and the lateral joint surfaces are examined with varus stress applied to the joint and the knee in almost complete extension. We have found that the different shape of the lateral tibial plateau and the greater rigidity of the lateral joint structures require 10−20° of flexion to allow the best possible visualization. Other authors have described the use of varus stress by applying pressure on the medial aspect of the joint at 90° of flexion (figure 4 position). In a healthy knee, the popliteal muscle can rarely be visual-

ized from inside the lateral joint space and has to be examined separately.

8. *Hiatus popliteus (lateral recess)*. The popliteal tendon perforates the posterior part of the lateral meniscus. Due to the tightness of the lateral joint space, inspection from a posterolateral approach is rarely possible, and it is necessary to advance the arthroscope laterally along the anterior horn of the meniscus or through the suprapatellar pouch. It is important to have the joint in extension and to open it by applying a valgus stress. Under these conditions, the tendon can be visualized satisfactorily at its perforation site through the meniscus. The hiatus popliteus is known to collect debris and should always be included in the arthroscopic examination.

9. *The posterior compartments*. The central approach is oriented towards the intercondylar notch and permits examination of the posterior compartments of the knee joint in most cases (Fig. **51**). With the knee hanging down, the cruciate ligament and the lateral side of the medial femoral condyle are visualized, and with slight pressure, the scope is then advanced posteriorly parallel to the tibial plateau. Medial rotation of the tibia may be necessary to allow easy passage of the arthroscope. However, if significant resistance is encountered, examination of the posterior joint compartment should be omitted. Distension and irrigation are important for examination of the posterior compartment. By rotating the instrument and changing to the 70° scope, the posterior capsule, the base of the posterior horn of the medial meniscus, the posterior aspect of the femoral condyle and the posterior part of the synovial lining of the posterior cruciate ligament can be inspected.
The posterolateral joint compartment can be examined in the same fashion. This compartment is more difficult to reach because the surgeon must negotiate past the anterior cruciate ligament and its tibial attachment. The posterior horn of the lateral meniscus, and occasionally the popliteal tendon can be inspected from the posterolateral approach. Access to the posterior compartments is facilitated in the presence of ligamentous instability or the absence of the cruciate ligaments. As the scope is withdrawn from the posterior joint compartments, the femoral attachments of both cruciate ligaments can be examined with the 70° scope (anterior cruciate from the lateral side, posterior cruciate from the medial side).

10. *Suprapatellar space: termination of the arthroscopy*. Diagnostic arthroscopy is concluded by bringing the instrument into the superior recess and visualizing the outflow cannula. Fixed or loose bodies and debris may have to be removed from this area; otherwise, these particles will remain in the periarticular tissues and cause disturbances of joint function.

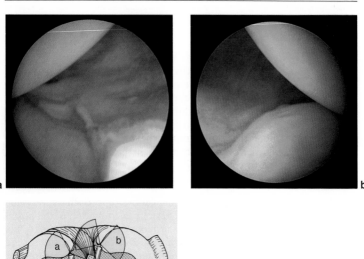

Fig. **51** Using the 70° scope, the posterolateral and posteromedial compartments can be visualized by way of transligamentous approach (**a, b**). By turning the 70° scope, the posterior cruciate ligament with its tibial insertion can be visualized (**c**)

Aspiration and synovial biopsy should be performed routinely in all arthroscopic examinations.

The diagnostic route is illustrated in Figure **52.** During arthroscopy, it is advisable to bear in mind not only the individual steps but the entire diagnostic route, as well. This helps to avoid such mistakes as termination of the arthroscopy after a positive pathological finding and thus overlooking a second lesion.

The transition from arthrotomy to arthroscopy requires adjustment and adaptation on the part of the surgeon. It is more difficult to judge the size of arthroscopically visualized objects and their spatial relationships due to the round visual field of the scope. Working inside a joint cavity causes one to lose orientation toward the body surface as well.

The location of the scope inside the joint depends multidimensionally on its own movements as well as on the position of the joint itself. Moreover, varus and valgus stress applied to the joint allow inspection

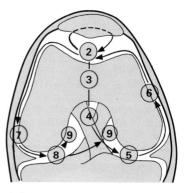

Fig. **52** Systematic approach to diagnostic arthroscopy of the knee. The arthroscopic examination should be performed in a systematic manner to allow visualization of all compartments of the joint. The joint should be in the following positions to facilitate the examination: (for 1st and 10th steps, see Fig. **50**)

2. suprapatellar:	hyperextended	no stress
3. trochlear groove:	increasing flexion	no stress
4. central:	30−90° of flexion	no stress
5. medial:	20−70° of flexion	valgus stress
6. peripheral:	30−50° of flexion	no stress
7. lateral gutter:	almost extended	valgus stress
8. lateral:	almost extended	varus stress
9. posterior:	90° of flexion	no stress

of joint compartments that usually cannot be seen during arthroscopy. The fact that large areas of the joint can be inspected often indicates pathological instability. For example, the medial compartment can often be visualized from the central approach without any additional maneuvers when the anterior cruciate ligament is ruptured and the medial collateral ligament is unstable.

All unexpected findings in the joint require evaluation of all other factors involved to explain the unclear situation.

On the other hand, rigid ligaments, which are often present in male patients, can make arthroscopic examination very difficult. If the femoral condyles are broad and flat, inspection of the lateral and posterior compartments carries an increased risk of damage to articular cartilage, especially in inexperienced hands. General anesthesia with additional pharmacological relaxation is sometimes helpful in the case of a patient with a very tight joint. However, except for knees which have been previously operated on and knees with osteoarthritis, there is no such thing as "a knee that is too tight."

The mechanics of the knee joint can be used to the surgeon's advantage to visualize certain structures, for example, the posterior horn of the medial meniscus can be examined much better with the 70° scope directed at the base of the posterior horn while the tibia is rotated internally.

The tendon of the popliteal muscle in the lateral joint space can only be visualized adequately by rotating the tibia in a contralateral direction. If the surgeon does not take advantage of these mechanical aids, an adequate statement cannot be made about the popliteal tendon.

Occasionally, routine preoperative X-rays will forecast difficulties in performing the arthroscopic procedure (Fig. **45**).

Severe degenerative joint disease with multiple osteophytes, osteocartilaginous spurs and structural changes can make arthroscopy difficult if not impossible. The central approach cannot be used in the presence of a patella baja, and a more medial approach must be chosen. Prior

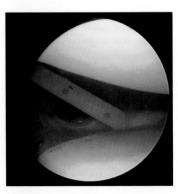

Fig. **53**   Normal arthroscopic findings: suprapatellar recess

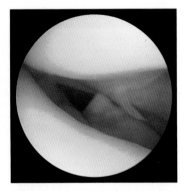

Fig. **54**   Normal arthroscopic findings: undersurface of the patella from distal approach

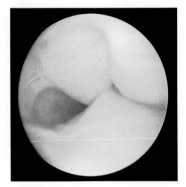

Fig. **55**   Normal arthroscopic findings: lateral recessus with view of hiatus popliteus

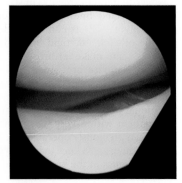

Fig. **56**   Normal arthroscopic findings: overview of the lateral joint compartment

surgery can alter the joint cavity severely and may force the arthroscopist to remodel the joint appropriately by shaving, or to abandon arthroscopy altogether.

The same is true for posttraumatic conditions in which intra-articular adhesions, osteophytes, as well as synovial reactions cause narrowing of the joint space.

The compartments visualized during diagnostic arthroscopy appear relatively homogeneous, as long as they are healthy joint structures. The different compartments are shown in Figures 53—60.

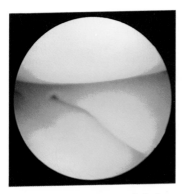

Fig. 57   Normal arthroscopic findings: overview of the medial joint compartment

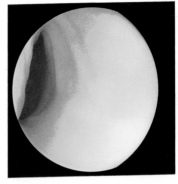

Fig. 58   Normal arthroscopic findings: medial recess with medial collateral ligament

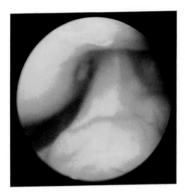

Fig. 59   Normal arthroscopic findings: intercondylar notch with anterior cruciate ligament

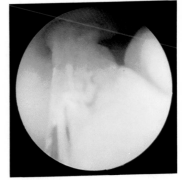

Fig. 60   Normal arthroscopic findings: anterior joint space with ligamentum mucosum

Examination of the Menisci

The meniscus consists of bradytrophic cartilage tissue with a central area of nutritional deficiency which may lead to degenerative changes and structural disorders. Any trauma or prolonged occupational stress can lead to lesions which always occur in the direction of the collagenous fibers. Since these fibers are arranged in an arcade-like pattern, different types of tears can result (vertical, horizontal, or radial tears, or longitudinal, bucket handle, or flap tears).

The primary lesion is usually a small longitudinal tear in the posterior horn which can extend and eventually result in total displacement of the torn fragment.

The different types of tears have been classified by Trillat (Fig. **61**).

Traumatic meniscus lesions are very common. Approximately 60 meniscectomies are performed annually per 100 000 persons. Meniscus lesions are three times more common in men than in women; the medial meniscus is affected in 80% of all cases, the lateral meniscus in 20%.

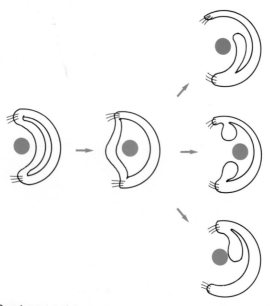

Fig. **61**   Development of the different tears in the meniscus beginning from a degenerative primary tear near the base and advancing to a complete bucket handle or flap tear in different cross-sections (blue spot indicates point of contact between femur and tibia)

The location of the meniscus lesion is determined by the occupational or athletic activity. Basketball injuries account for right-sided meniscus lesions in approximately 80% of the injuries; in wrestlers, the lateral meniscus is injured in 45% of all cases.

These empirical facts should be taken into consideration in the evaluation of a painful knee. Knowledge of frequency and incidence of these injuries aids in the differential diagnosis.

The symptoms of a meniscus lesion are variable. A fresh, trapped bucket handle tear usually results in a locked knee with effusion or hemarthrosis and an inability to bear weight on the affected extremity. The diagnosis is not difficult; concurrent injuries must be ruled out. A slowly progressing degenerative lesion of the posterior horn, on the other hand, has different and less characteristic clinical symptoms.

Since arthroscopy is both a diagnostic and a therapeutic procedure, the decision to schedule a patient for arthroscopy is often made without a thorough clinical examination and exact operative indication. This seems to be a general problem. Very few arthroscopists can resist the temptation to look into the joint, especially since other diagnostic modalities are not without risk and are time-consuming as well. These procedures are less accurate than arthroscopy and do not have the option to conclude the diagnostic study with the appropriate surgical procedure.

Arthrography has a diagnostic accuracy of approximately 85%, but it does not allow an arthroscopic procedure to be performed for at least 14 days (synovitis, risk of infection).

Computed tomography, even with contrast, suffers from a poor diagnostic accuracy for the menisci. The resolution of MRI has to be improved significantly to achieve sufficient visualization of the surfaces of the menisci in order to make decisions about the need for possible surgery.

Clinical examination remains the most important diagnostic modality for making a decision about meniscectomy. The symptoms are provoked during examination by simulating motion, compression, and rotation, thus inducing stress on the knee. Nevertheless, the clinical history alone often leads to arthroscopy. This is particularly true for recurrent joint-locking due to loose bodies or a bucket handle tear of the meniscus.

Arthroscopic Diagnosis of the Menisci

Meniscus Tears: Types, Locations, and Examination

All meniscal tears can be reduced to three basic types (longitudinal, radial, horizontal), which occur with different frequency in the medial and lateral menisci. As a result of the anatomic location of the lateral meniscus, tears can occur in specific locations. Since the basic diagnosis do not differ otherwise, both the medial and the lateral meniscal tears are discussed together. The medial meniscus is directly attached to the collateral ligament which makes it more susceptible to tears since it is less mobile and cannot avoid being trapped (80% of all tears involve the medial meniscus). Degenerative tears resulting from chronic abuse are also more common in the medial than in the lateral posterior horn.

The palpation of the menisci is done in the following manner: With the tip pointed upward, the probing hook is moved from peripheral to central over the body of the meniscus to test consistency and stability of the meniscus. In addition, the interface between capsule and meniscus should be tested with the probing hook. After that, the edge of the meniscus is lifted up, the undersurface is inspected, an attemot is made to pull the meniscus into the joint with the hook to test for tissue weakness and possible longitudinal tears. The posterior horn should be carefully inspected, as most of the tears occur there. Typical meniscus tears are illustrated in Figure **62** for the medial meniscus.

Longitudinal Tears

1. The undisplaced type. This tear is most commonly seen in the posterior horn but can extend to the middle and anterior parts of the meniscus. Isolated longitudinal tears of the anterior horn are rare. They are more common in the lateral meniscus, but have little clinical significance. A longitudinal tear can occur at any level of the meniscus, either in the avascular area or in the area close to the capsule; occasionally it involves both parts. A tear in the avascular part is usually degenerative, while a tear close to the capsule is generally a traumtic lesion. It is often associated with an injury of the anterior cruciate ligament. Incomplete tears are seen occasionally; they occur most

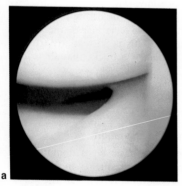 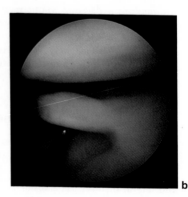

a   b

Fig. **62 a + b**

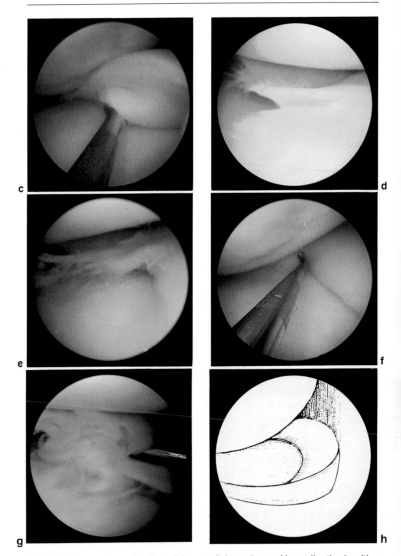

Fig. 62 Diagnostic evaluation of the medial meniscus. Normally, the healthy meniscus has a smooth surface, continous contours and a firm connection with the capsule (**a**). The most commonly occuring tears are flap tears (**b**), bucket handle tears (**c**), and radial tears (**d**). The common degeneration of the posterior horn (**e**) is sometimes not immediately evident (**f**). The probing hook helps to pull the destroyed part of the meniscus into the joint space (**g**). The schematic drawing (**h**) illustrates these examples

commonly on the undersurface of the meniscus. The resulting instability can be tested with the probing hook. Occasionally, an incomplete longitudinal tear may connect with a horizontal tear, indicating beginning degeneration.

An undisplaced tear close to the capsule can sometimes be overlooked since the actual tear is not in the field of vision, and the meniscus appears superficially normal. Testing for mobility with the hook is of particular importance in these cases. The tear itself can be visualized during introduction of the arthroscope into the posterolateral or posteromedial compartment.

A tear close to the capsule at the hiatus popliteus is unique to the lateral meniscus and can extend anteriorly as well as posteriorly. Routine examination of the recessus popliteus is therefore of great importance during diagnostic arthroscopy.

Depending on the length of the tear, the meniscus may or may not be displaced and can even be found in the intercondylar notch (tears of more than 3 cm in length).

2. The dislocated type (bucket handle tear). A bucket handle tear may present diagnostic problems because the peripheral rim resembles a degenerated meniscus and the "bucket handle" in the intercondylar notch may be overlooked.

Occasionally, the dislocated bucket handle makes inspection of the involved compartment difficult, especially for the inexperienced surgeon and may cause him to miss the diagnosis. Inability to visualize a compartment should always raise the suspicion that a bucket handle tear is present. To document the extent of the tear, the dislocated bucket handle should be repositioned with the probing hook, which is also the first step for its excision.

3. Flap tear. This tear is a combination of a longitudinal and a radial tear. It is usually found as a simple flap tear but can appear as a double flap tear after division of the bridge of a bucket handle tear. It is usually attached anteriorly, since the tissue bridge of a longitudinal tear is more prone to rupture at the posterior horn.

Flap tears can also occur as a component of a horizontal tear in one of the two parts. This particular situation can cause diagnostic problems when the tear is located under the body of the meniscus at the edge of the tibial plateau where it cannot easily be seen. In other cases, the tear may be superior and lateral in the capsular area and can be identified without difficulty. It is of great importance to examine the edge of a suspicious-looking meniscus with a probing hook for possible flap tears. A posteromedially or posterolaterally displaced flap tear can only be identified if both of these compartments are inspected carefully. A pedicled flap with base in the anterior horn can complicate arthroscopic orientation in the joint from a central approach because of its proximity to the arthroscope and may only be identified after considerable search.

Radial Tears

A radial tear is typical for the lateral meniscus. It usually occurs in the middle third and should not present any diagnostic problems. In some cases, the two edges slide into each other and the tear can only be verified after careful palpation.

Horizontal Tears

This tear is typical for a degenerated meniscus and occurs most commonly in combination with a flap tear or with generalized destruction or fraying of the entire meniscus.

The posterior horn of the medial meniscus is the most frequent localization of horizontal tears. They are an indication of degeneration and vascular insufficiency of the meniscus, and the tear often extends to the capsule. In the lateral meniscus, a cyst can often be found in combination with a horizontal tear. Occasionally, a gelatinous substance escapes from the orifice of the cyst into the joint when pressure is applied to the cyst. If the orifice cannot be identified, a needle can be directed from the outside through the cyst into the joint as an aid in establishing the spatial relationship between the cyst and the meniscus. Careful examination with the hook is necessary to document the extent of cartilage destruction and the presence of a cyst. As mentioned above, a horizontal tear can present as a flap tear with all the diagnostic difficulties associated with this lesion. In rare cases, a horizontal tear combined with a longitudinal tear can appear as a double bucket handle tear.

Hiatus Popliteus

The hiatus popliteus in the lateral meniscus is an anatomical peculiarity. The tendon of the popliteal muscle penetrates the lateral meniscus and is covered by synovial membrane. The popliteal muscle stabilizes the knee in rotation but can accomplish this only as long as the hiatus in the lateral meniscus is well preserved. This must be taken into account during diagnostic and operative arthroscopy (Figs. **63, 64**).

Discoid Meniscus

The discoid meniscus can be considered a variant or a developmental abnormality. It is rarely found on the medial side, more often laterally (Fig. **65**).

The transition from a normal to a discoid meniscus is gradual, from a broad meniscus to a discoid structure that extends into the intercondylar notch; the edges of the meniscus cannot be seen. At first glance, one might suspect that the meniscus is absent. Palpation of the tibial plateau which is covered with the discoid meniscus, however, allows one to make the diagnosis quickly. Tears of the discoid meniscus can be identified without difficulty. Incomplete but symptomatic tears on the

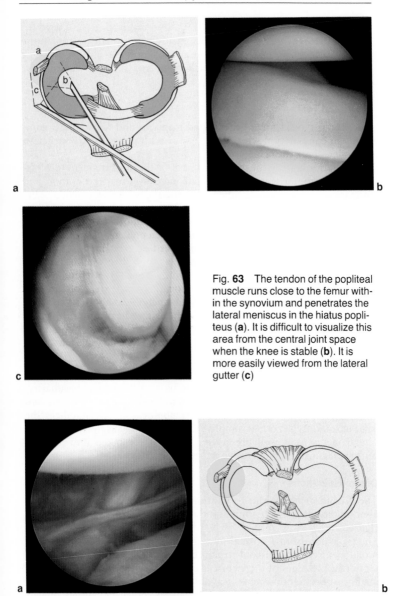

Fig. **63** The tendon of the popliteal muscle runs close to the femur within the synovium and penetrates the lateral meniscus in the hiatus popliteus (**a**). It is difficult to visualize this area from the central joint space when the knee is stable (**b**). It is more easily viewed from the lateral gutter (**c**)

Fig. **64** Resection of the lateral meniscus has to be done carefully, preserving those parts of the meniscus that form the hiatus popliteus (subtotal resection)

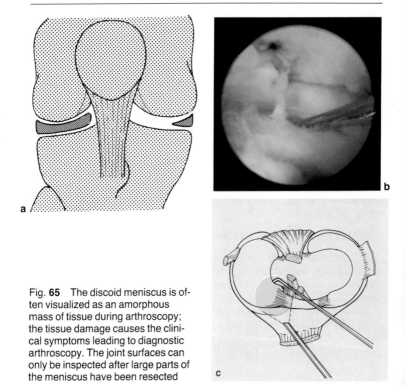

Fig. **65**   The discoid meniscus is often visualized as an amorphous mass of tissue during arthroscopy; the tissue damage causes the clinical symptoms leading to diagnostic arthroscopy. The joint surfaces can only be inspected after large parts of the meniscus have been resected

undersurface, however, cannot be visualized in this situation. The probing hook should be used to examine the meniscus carefully. A soft spot should raise the suspicion that a tear is present. A bucket handle tear in a discoid meniscus can cause considerable diagnostic problems and may be difficult to excise because of its size.

In summary it should be pointed out that careful examination with the probing hook of every meniscus, regardless of how normal it may appear, is mandatory since tears in the hidden parts of the meniscus can only be diagnosed by indirect signs such as hypermobility or displacement. Even if the tear can be seen easily, examination with the probing hook is important in order to document the extent of the rupture. Posterolateral and posteromedial compartments should be examined with the tibia in different positions of rotation to allow detection of tears in these areas. If a tear is found, the other meniscus should still be examined since bilateral meniscus tears are not uncommon, especially when anterior and posterior cruciate ligament ruptures are present as well.

Exact inspection and palpation of both menisci in their entirety as well as their insertion sites at the capsule make the arthroscopic examination complete.

Examination of Capsule and Ligaments

Diagnostic workup of capsule and ligaments is based on clinical examination; arthroscopy is usually used to confirm the findings obtained by history, clinical examination and tests for stability (if necessary under anesthesia). In certain situations, however, arthroscopy may be necessary to establish the correct diagnosis.

Clinical Examination of Capsule and Ligaments

The knee joint moves in several different planes. The interrelationships of the various stabilizing functions are known. Loss of a single ligament can, under certain circumstances, be compensated by other fibrous or muscular elements of the joint.

Prior to arthroscopy, the following tests should be performed routinely even if there is no suspicion of a ligament lesion (Fig. **66**):

1. drawer test in 20° of flexion (Lachman test),
2. varus and valgus stress tests in extension,
3. varus and valgus stress tests in 30° of flexion,
4. anterior drawer test in internal and external rotation with the knee in 90° of flexion,
5. posterior drawer test,
6. pivot shift test and, if necessary, its variations.

When these tests are performed correctly in the painfree and relaxed patient, the results generally allow an exact documentation of the stability of the knee joint.

In cases of fresh trauma, or if the patient is unable to relax completely, the examination should be done under anesthesia. In appropriate cases, a conservative treatment plan can be initiated after these tests have been done. We are of the opinion that arthroscopic examination should be performed in all cases once the patient has agreed to an examination under anesthesia. The additional information gained by inspection of the joint surfaces can be very valuable and in the patient's interest (simultaneous lesions of meniscus and articular cartilage!).

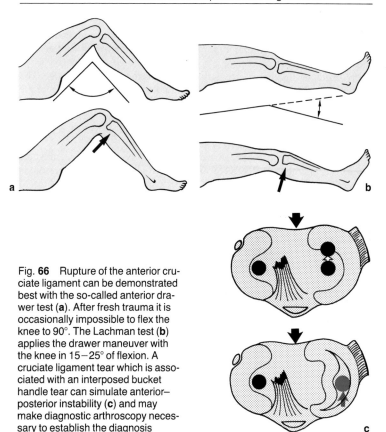

Fig. **66** Rupture of the anterior cruciate ligament can be demonstrated best with the so-called anterior drawer test (**a**). After fresh trauma it is occasionally impossible to flex the knee to 90°. The Lachman test (**b**) applies the drawer maneuver with the knee in 15–25° of flexion. A cruciate ligament tear which is associated with an interposed bucket handle tear can simulate anterior–posterior instability (**c**) and may make diagnostic arthroscopy necessary to establish the diagnosis

Arthroscopic Evaluation of Capsular and Ligamentous Structures

(Fig. **67**)

Most injuries to joint capsule and ligaments require immediate evaluation. This should be done as an acute arthroscopic procedure with the option of immediate repair of the damaged joint structures. Chronic instability can be clarified by clinical examination in most cases and diagnostic arthroscopy or examination under anesthesia are usually not necessary. However, because of the high incidence of articular cartilage and meniscus lesions found in association with chronic instability, arthroscopy may be useful before reconstructive surgery of the ligaments is scheduled.

Both cruciate ligaments are palpated with the probing hook. The posterior cruciate ligament is best examined with the 70° scope from the posteromedial approach. The femoral insertion sites of the anterior and posterior cruciate ligaments are seen with the 70° scope (pointed upward) as the scope is slowly pulled out of the posterolateral and posteromedial compartments, respectively.

If a subsynovial rupture is suspected, the synovial envelope must be opened to examine the ligamentous fibers. In all other cases, pressure is applied to the ligament with the probing hook to test its tension. If tension seems to be reduced, the examination is repeated while the drawer test is applied at the same time. In cases of old ruptures with rotatory instability, mobility of the joint is best demonstrated in the posterior compartments where the femoral condyles are observed as they slide and rotate over the posterior horns of the menisci during the drawer and rotatory provocation tests.

The collateral ligaments can only be evaluated indirectly, for example, severe rotatory instability can be an indication for the existence of a collateral ligament lesion (Fig. **68**). At the same time, the ipsilateral compartment usually opens up wider and can be visualized better than in a normal joint. In an acute rupture, part of the collateral ligament

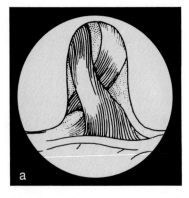

Fig. **67** Arthroscopic diagnosis of the cruciate ligaments. The intact cruciate ligament is under considerable tension and cannot be deformed with the probing hook (**a**). If it can be pulled into traction with the hook, it has to be considered elongated (**b**). The femoral insertion site at the medial aspect of the lateral condyle has to be checked. A missing or damaged insertion site (**c**) indicates an old tear. Sometimes the cruciate ligament is ruptured without concomitant injury of the synovia (**d**). If suspicion of a tear exists, the synovial cover needs to be opened and the collagen fibers have to be examined for evidence of a rupture (**e**). Hemorrhage can also occur subsynovially (**f**). More common is a complete splitting of the fibers (**g**)

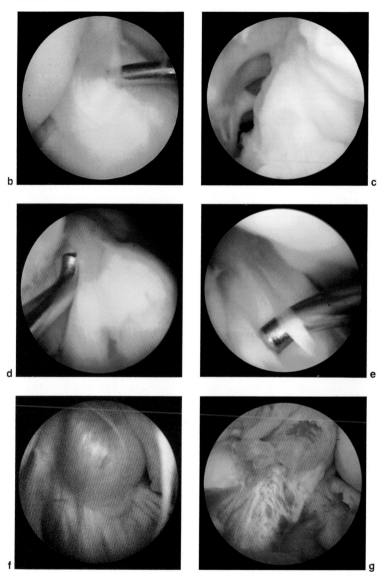

Fig. **67b—g**

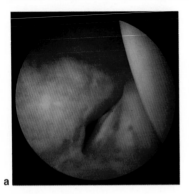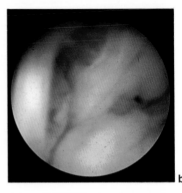

Fig. **68**   Arthroscopic capsule diagnosis. The arthroscopic signs for capsular lesions are fresh hemorrhage (**a**) that cause pain at palpation, and instability that can be demonstrated clinically as lateral instability (**b**)

may be folded into the joint and a rupture of the joint capsule may be visible.

The menisci are located in the immediate vicinity of the ligaments and can be used to determine the location of the rupture (tibial or femoral). If the meniscus is pulled upward, the collateral ligament is usually torn at its tibial insertion.

The importance of a careful history and physical examination cannot be stressed enough. Some surgical procedures have proved to be unnecessary and could have been avoided if appropriate care had been taken preoperatively. It should be kept in mind that arthroscopy is an invasive procedure which opens the joint cavity. It should not be taken lightly and should be used only when indicated.

Evaluation of Articular Cartilage and Patella

Examination of Articular Cartilage

Cartilage is a bradytrophic tissue which derives its nutrition from the subchondral bone and the joint fluid. It is attached to the bone by special fiber systems. Cartilage can sustain significant stresses—especially shearing forces—due to its unique surface design, provided it is lubricated appropriately.

Damage to the articular surface can be easily recognized during arthroscopy. According to Fründ and Outerbridge, these lesions can be classified into three categories (Fig. **69**):

Fig. **69** Classification according to Fründ and Outerbridge. Grade 1 refers to minor irregularities of the cartilage and edematous swelling. In grade 2 clefts are visible within the cartilage, which extend down to the bone in grade 3 and partially expose the bone. The drawings **a—c** illustrate this classification. These changes cannot be identified on plain X-rays. Diagnostic confirmation is only possible by direct (arthroscopic) visualization (Figs. **d—f**)

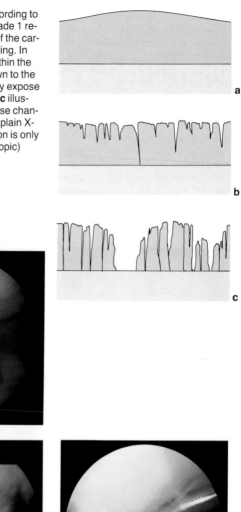

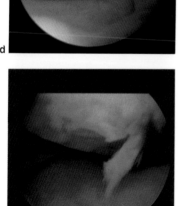

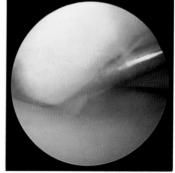

Grade 1 refers to softening and edematous swelling of the cartilage with an increase in thickness.

Grade 2 is characterized by a loss of structural integrity and destruction of the smooth surface which does not extend to the bone.

Grade 3 refers to a complete loss of structure with detachment of the cartilage from the bone or the formation of cartilage clefts extending down to the bone.

Arthroscopic examination of the articular cartilage includes evaluation of color as well as consistency of the cartilage, which is tested by probing with the hook. If the tip of the hook can be pressed into the cartilage without leaving any traces, grade 1 is diagnosed.

Clefts and fraying detected with the hook signify a grade 2 lesion.

If the cartilage can be lifted up from the bone with the instrument or the tip of the instrument scratches the surface of the bone, grade 3 damage is present.

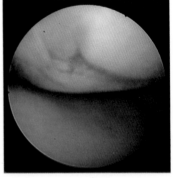

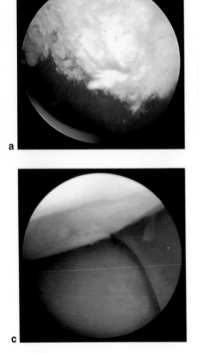

Fig. **70** Pathological changes in articular cartilage surfaces. Typical surface changes can be found in gouty arthritis (**a**), deepening of the cartilage in osteochondritis dissecans (**b**), and the formation of pannus in inflammatory rheumatic disease (**c**)

These changes can also be documented by computed tomography using additional contrast media. However, therapeutic measures cannot be undertaken immediately after CT, in contrast to diagnostic arthroscopy.

Typical pathological findings (Fig. **70**) are the various degrees of chondromalacia with reactive pannus, osteochondritis dissecans, or crystalline deposits in the course of diverse metabolic diseases.

Examination of the Patella
(Fig. **71**)

The cartilaginous undersurface of the patella can be involved in general degenerative changes of cartilage according to Fründ's classification, but it may also be damaged by other specific mechanical causes which can be best summarized as imbalances of forces during walking. A weak quadriceps muscle, abnormal valgus deformity of the knee joint with a change in the Q-angle, or a dysplasia of one of the two articulating surfaces may be at fault. Arthroscopy is the best suited diagnostic test for these problems and should focus on testing the alignment of the patella during different degress of flexion. The distention of the joint does not have to be taken into consideration, as it has been found that even with elevated pressure in the joint space the degree of lateralization remains unchanged. According to the findings, the arthroscopy may again be followed by immediate repair.

Besides the status of the cartilage and the alignment, the two facets of the patella have to be examined for acute or chronic changes which may be induced by traumatic or recurrent dislocation of the patella.

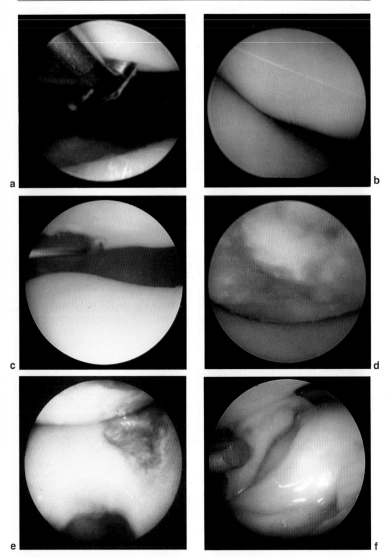

Fig. **71** Underside of the patella and the trochlear groove. The consistency of the cartilage on the underside of the patella is tested (**a**). Occasionally edematous swellings (**b**), loss of tissue structure (**c**), or considerable ulceration (**d**) are observed. Ulceration of the trochlear groove (**e**) or postarthroscopic injuries (**f**) can be seen

Disorders of the Synovial Membrane and Plica Syndrome

Disorders of the Synovium

The synovial lining of the knee joint (Fig. **72**) should routinely be examined during arthroscopy. We take a synovial biopsy in each case. Arthroscopy and exact examination of the synovium of the knee joint may be indicated for a wide variety of symptoms and diseases.

The appearance of the synovium may vary depending on the course of the examination, the distention of the joint, the use of a tourniquet, the time that has elapsed since a preceding arthrography, and so on. An exact description cannot be given. Experience will enable the examiner to diagnose certain conditions from the appearance of the synovium.

Synovial changes resulting from inflammatory conditions like rheuma-

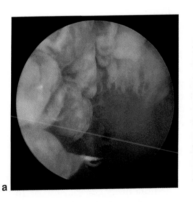

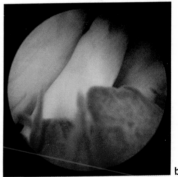

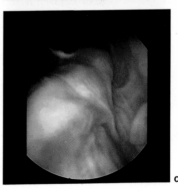

Fig. **72** Synovial pathology. Depending on the intra-articular pressure and the pressure of the tourniquet, the normal synovium shows more or less pronounced vascular markings. In nonspecific synovitis, many grass-like villi (**a**) and pronounced vascular injection are seen. Accompanying synovitis is defined as an irritation of the synovium in the presence of another pathological condition, here a bucket handle tear (**b**). More pronounced changes are seen in synovitis villonodularis (**c**)

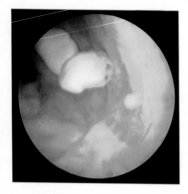

Fig. **73**   Synovial chondromatosis.
Cartilaginous hypertrophy can occur, representing metaplastic
changes of the synovium. They occur as solitary or multiple chondral
formations which are attached to the
synovium initially and then become
free bodies. This can lead to tamponade of the joint

tic diseases, lupus erythematosus, ankylosing spondylitis, gout, and
infectious or viral diseases can be attributed to these conditions based
on the history alone.

In some cases, however, only arthroscopy leads to the correct diagnosis
(for example, synovitis caused by chlamydia infection).

Pigmented villonodular synovitis (Fig. **72c**) and synovial chondromatosis (Fig. **73**) are typical diseases of the synovial membrane. Both
conditions are metaplastic changes of the synovium. Pigmented villonodular synovitis forms tumors of the synovial lining which frequently
cause swelling of the knee. Synovial chondromatosis is characterized by
a proliferation of small cartilaginous bodies the size of rice kernels
which grow in the joint and can cause tamponade of the entire joint
space in extreme cases.

A special type of damage is seen in hemophiliacs; neoplasms of the
synovium should also be considered in the differential diagnosis. Much
more common, however, are non-specific reactions of the synovium
which may result in a bizarre appearance which is often confusing to the
beginner in diagnostic arthroscopy, especially after prior surgery or
other damage to the joint.

A detailed outline of histopathological findings in the synovial membrane can be found in the publications of Klein and Huth (1980).

Plica Syndrome

The plica synovialis medialis hypertrophicans represents an anatomical
variation. It is of pathological significance because it can damage the
articular cartilage of the femoral condyle (Fig. **74**).

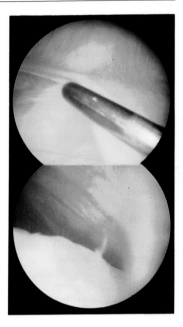

Fig. **74** Plica shelf syndrome. This is characterized by hypertrophy of the plica synovialis medialis (of unknown etiology) that causes damage of the articular cartilage of the medial femoral condyle, resulting in snapping phenomena

Arthroscopy in Acute Trauma

Every traumatic hemarthrosis, especially in young and active patients, should be evaluated by arthroscopy within two weeks if radiological studies do not reveal the cause. Even if the X-rays show fractures, diagnostic arthroscopy may be of value in certain cases (bone and cartilage lesions after dislocation of the patella, fractures of the tibial plateau and the intercondylar eminence). The commonly practiced examination of the knee under anesthesia, in our opinion, is not sufficient, as certain lesions (for example, bucket handle tear of the meniscus associated with a cruciate ligament rupture) may be overlooked.

Furthermore, knowledge of the exact extent of the intra-articular damage is of great importance when the patient's rehabilitation is planned, especially as far as early mobilization and weight-bearing is concerned. The operation should be performed within two weeks from the time of the injury, as the repair of certain lesions, such as ruptured ligaments and meniscus detachments, probably yields better results when performed within that time period.

The following questions must be answered during arthroscopy of acute injuries:

1. What is the source of the bleeding?
2. Is a meniscus tear present?
3. Can the torn meniscus be repaired or is meniscectomy necessary?
4. Are tendons or ligaments torn, and can they be repaired?
5. Are injuries to bone and cartilage present and can they be repaired?
6. Was the patella dislocated?

Acute arthroscopy should always be preceded by routine stability testing of the knee under anesthesia.

Since ruptures of the joint capsule or other lesions of the surrounding structures may have occurred with the knee injury, pressure of the irrigation fluid should be kept lower than normal to avoid extravasation and soft tissue edema. If the pressure is kept at approximately 100 mmHg, no significant extravasation of fluid will occur.

Arthroscopy should be avoided if the head of the fibula is fractured; compartment syndromes have been observed under these conditions.

The procedure is the same as that used for routine diagnostic arthroscopy. A leg holder, camera, and two arthroscopes are necessary. The roller pump is of particular help in acute arthroscopy, as the better irrigation allows for better visualization thereby shortening the examination time. The outflow cannula is also of special importance if the surgeon decides not to use the tourniquet for hemostasis. If bleeding continues, however, a tourniquet should be inflated to improve and shorten the irrigation time.

The arthroscopy is started by introducing a 30° arthroscope through a central approach. The outflow cannula is inserted into the suprapatellar recess from the lateral side. The cannula is initially kept open for irrigation of the joint and removal of blood clots. Using this technique, an irrigation of the joint prior to insertion of the arthroscope is not necessary. The roller pump is set at maximal flowrate with the outflow cannula wide open, thereby keeping the pressure in the joint minimal. If the pump is not pressure-controlled, the patency of the outflow cannula should be checked intermittently. Otherwise the procedure is the same as for routine diagnostic arthroscopy.

There are typical injuries that should be treated with arthroscopic surgery. Composition of the bloody fluid obtained from the joint allows some conclusions as to the type of injury. With a pure hemarthrosis, capsular or meniscus injuries can be expected; the presence of fat in the effusion raises the suspicion of an osteochondral fracture.

Osteochondral Lesions

Acute Dislocation of the Patella

At first glance, bleeding into the medial retinaculum is noted. When the patella is examined during flexion and extension, a tendency toward subluxation is found and in some cases a shearing fracture of the cartilage from the facets of the patella can be identified. In these cases it is important to examine the lateral femoral condyle in its entirety to rule out a corresponding shearing fracture. Depending on the size and extent of the fracture, it may be fixed arthroscopically or by way of arthro-tomy with tissue glue, wires, or screws. The fibrin adhesive is ineffective in cases of pure chondral fractures. In cases of smaller fractures in non–weight-bearing areas and pure chondral fractures, the loose body should be removed since pieces of cartilage usually do not heal properly. This concept is also valuable for fragments broken off the patellar surface.

Osteochondral Fracture

A fracture of cartilage and bone is most often the result of direct trauma and can occur at the medial and lateral femoral condyles as well as in the area of the patellar facets. Associated injuries of the ligaments and the menisci are common. Impression fractures without loose bodies do not need any specific treatment, while loose bodies need to be removed because it is difficult to fix them back into their original positions, and they heal very poorly.

Fracture of the Intercondylar Eminence

In these cases, arthroscopy is of diagnostic importance. The degree of dislocation and incongruity of the joint can be assessed and the tension of the anterior cruciate ligament can be tested by palpation. If the dislocation is minimal and the anterior cruciate ligament is intact, conservative treatment is feasible. If, however, the anterior cruciate ligament is incompetent, arthroscopic or open surgical fixation is mandatory.

Impression Fracture of the Tibial Plateau

In cases of incongruity of the tibial plateau, the congruity can be restored under arthroscopic visualization and loose fragments may be removed arthroscopically (Fig. **94**).

Lesions of Ligaments and Menisci

Anterior Cruciate Ligament Rupture and Medial Meniscus Tear

This is a combination injury commonly seen in contact sports like football or soccer. As opposed to old cruciate ligament ruptures, a fresh rupture can be overlooked, especially if it is subsynovial. Careful palpation with the probing hook and a provocation test (anterior drawer test) are of the utmost importance. The femoral insertion site should also be inspected carefully, which is accomplished best by inserting the arthroscope into the posterolateral compartment, switching then to the 70° scope, and slowly pulling the instrument back with the scope directed upward. Subsynovial bleeding is recognized by a dark appearance of the synovium and a change in the superficial vascular pattern. In these cases, the synovium should be opened and the ligament itself should be probed with the hook. The anterior drawer test reveals insufficient tension of the anterior cruciate ligament. The associated tear of the meniscus is often a longitudinal tear in the vascular portion (Fig. **67**) which is amenable to reconstructive (often arthroscopic) surgery, particulary in the younger patient. At the same time, the anterior cruciate ligament has to be sutured and strengthened. If the meniscus is generally of poor quality, however, it should be removed.

Anterior Cruciate Ligament and Collateral Ligament Rupture

This is one of the most common complex injuries and is associated with a tear in the medial meniscus in almost every case. The extent of the lesion of the medial collateral ligament can be assessed during examination under anesthesia. An associated rupture of the posterior oblique ligament can be diagnosed arthroscopically. The tear is usually in the tibial portion of the ligament and the meniscus is pulled up above the tibial plateau; it is usually shaped like a wave. Once the scope is moved under the meniscus and the tissues are palpated, an area of hemorrhage is often detected. Occasionally the ligament is folded into the joint. This type of injury requires surgical repair as soon as possible.

Posterior Cruciate Ligament Rupture in Combination with Detachment of the Medial or Lateral Meniscus

This combination is much rarer than those discussed above. The diagnosis of the posterior cruciate ligament rupture follows the same guidelines as given for the anterior cruciate ligament. It can also be present as a subsynovial rupture with intact synovium and the ligament may appear normal to inspection. The palpation with the hook from an almost central anterior or a posteromedial approach is of the greatest importance. The synovial sheath around the ligament should be opened.

The femoral insertion site of the ligament is found by pulling the arthroscope back from posteromedial to anteromedial with the 70° degree scope pointed upward. The posterior cruciate ligament rupture is sometimes combined with a detachment of the lateral meniscus in the area of the popliteal recess. The rupture of the lateral mensicus close to the capsule tends to heal very well and therefore, conservative treatment is indicated (cast for four weeks and no weight-bearing). After severe trauma to the posterolateral compartment, the popliteal tendon may be ruptured, which can be easily diagnosed arthroscopically. Surgical treatment is inevitable in those cases.

Other Lesions

Beyond the already discussed lesions, any combination of meniscal tears including degenerative tears either isolated or with cruciate or other ligament ruptures can be found during acute arthroscopy. Of particular interest is the crash rupture of the lateral or medial posterior horn after severe trauma which represents a comminuted rupture of an otherwise young and healthy meniscus requiring meniscectomy.

Associated findings, sometimes even isolated, are capsule ruptures in the posterolateral or posteromedial compartments which are not of prognostic significance if they are not combined with a cruciate ligament rupture.

In some cases the damage and the source of bleeding cannot be detected during acute arthroscopy.

In general, diagnostic arthroscopy helps to determine the plan for conservative or surgical treatment.

Ruptured collateral ligaments with minimal instability require immediate immobilization without weight-bearing for four weeks, provided no concomitant instability of the cruciate ligaments is present. Ruptured cruciate ligaments in athletically active patients are treated surgically according to general orthopedic principles, as conservative treatment often results in instability, which may force the patient to give up certain sports (for example, soccer). Isolated tears of the anterior cruciate ligament can be treated conservatively if the patient is not very active, as the resulting instability is minimal and does not pose a problem in everyday life. Combination injuries represent a therapeutic dilemma (collateral and anterior cruciate ligament). Elderly patients may be treated conservatively but younger patients with athletic interests should undergo surgical treatment for both ligaments to provide maximal stability.

Arthroscopic Surgery

Survey of Indications, Prerequisites, and Techniques

The following indications for operative arthroscopy have been developed so far:

- meniscectomy,
- removal of loose bodies,
- refixation of osteochondral lesions and pridie drilling,
- cartilage abrasion and removal of osteophytes,
- synovectomy, lysis of adhesions,
- meniscus repair,
- reconstruction of cruciate ligaments.

Some of these methods are still in the developmental stage. In the future, however, all surgical procedures on the surfaces of the joint will be done endoscopically.

The axiom which states that a good open procedure is better than a poorly executed closed procedure is still in the best interest of the patient. Great potential for iatrogenic injuries to the knee exist alongside the obvious advantages of the endoscopic procedure, particularly during the learning phase of this new technique. In contrast to diagnostic arthroscopy, operative arthroscopy should always be done under general anesthesia. The procedure itself is principally the same: a leg holder, an irrigation system, a video camera, and two arthroscopes are required.

Instruments for hand use and powered tools are offered in a large variety. The minimum requirement in equipment is listed on page 40. This list can be extended according to interest and the experience of the individual surgeon.

A tourniquet is routinely placed around the thigh and is only inflated if necessary during the operation.

A thorough examination of the knee under anesthesia is imperative prior to arthroscopic surgery. First the leg is lifted from the leg holder to produce the pivot-shift maneuver. Next, varus and valgus stress, the Lachmann test, and drawer tests are performed.

The central approach is most useful for operative arthroscopic procedures. In general, the 30° scope is used, but occasionally for procedures on the anterior horn and in the posterior compartments, the 70° scope may be necessary.

A requirement for successful arthroscopic surgery is the ability of the surgeon to use the different instruments both with the right and the left hand. Both left- and right-handed persons can achieve this capability in a short time by practicing on a model.

Meniscus Surgery

Diagnostic evaluation of the entire knee joint should be completed before resection or repair of the meniscus is started. Evaluation with the probing hook is important in assessing the extent of the damage to the meniscus prior to its resection. There are no major differences between surgery on the medial and the lateral meniscus and therefore, the described techniques are applicable to both sides barring some exceptions.

Longitudinal Tear, Undisplaced Type

The extent of the tear is first assessed with the probing hook and then the posterior aspect of the tear is visualized. An ipsilateral portal is used for introducing a straight basket forceps. If the posterior horn is difficult to reach, a small basket forceps with a short, upward-bent tip is used and the dorsal bridge of the tear is resected until only a thin layer of tissue is left. The posterior horn can then be trimmed with the same instrument, leaving a smooth transition to the remaining meniscus rim after resection of the meniscus. The part of the meniscus to be resected should be fixed to the tibial plateau with a needle which is introduced from the outside to the inside to avoid losing the fragment after it is resected and freely mobile within the joint. Then the anterior tissue bridge may be transected, which is done best via a superior contralateral portal with the straight or upward-bent basket forceps. Tears that extend into the anterior horn can often be reached with a 60°-angled scissors through an ipsilateral approach. The anterior tissue bridge is then transected. The channel for the extraction of the fragment is then enlarged in all directions at the skin and subcutaneous levels before extraction is attempted to avoid losing the fragment in the channel. The largest possible grasping forceps is introduced and the meniscus is grasped at the anterior edge of the resection so that the forceps and the meniscus fragment are in one line. After the transfixing needle has been removed, the fragment is extracted under constant rotational movements through the channel. This can be facilitated by grasping the fragment in the channel with a Kocher clamp. Then the remaining meniscus is examined for rough edges, tears, and free particles. If present, these areas should be resected or smoothed using a straight basket forceps in the area of the posterior horn and a 90° basket forceps in the middle aspect. For rough areas in the anterior horn, the 90°-

angled basket forceps is introduced from superior contralateral (3 cm from the midline and 3 cm above the arthroscope). It is important to leave at least a 2 mm tissue bridge of the lateral meniscus in front of the popliteal tendon since a complete removal of the meniscus here results in instability. This rule applies to all procedures done on the lateral meniscus. If, in the case of an incomplete longitudinal rupture, the decision has been made to resect the meniscus, this should be done using the straight basket forceps for the posterior horn and the 90°-angled basket forceps in the middle part, both from an ipsilateral approach. The more elegant surgery using scalpel or scissors should only be attempted by an experienced surgeon. Resection of the meniscus at the anterior horn can be commenced in the corresponding manner (Figs. **75**, **76**).

Bucket Handle Tear

This tear is most commonly found in young athletic patients and is seen in the medial meniscus in 90% of the cases. The same rules apply as for the dislocated rupture (Figs. **75** and **76**). After the diagnosis is established, the next step is the repositioning of the bucket handle and resection according to the principles of resection for longitudinal ruptures. In exceptional cases with longstanding symptoms prior to surgery, repositioning sometimes proves to be impossible. In these cases the posterior horn is resected from a superior contralateral approach (tissue bridge!); the anterior part of the rupture is resected from the same approach using a basket forceps or hooked scissors, or, in the case of an ipsilateral approach, with angled scissors. The extraction is done as described above. A bucket handle tear is also called a dislocated longitudinal tear, which means that the free part will intermittently or permanently block the joint by falling into the central intercondylar compartment.

This type of tear is often associated with a synovitis which limits the intra-articular visibility. In such cases, a partial synovectomy should be performed first (with power instruments), to improve visualization since meniscectomy with inadequate visibility is usually unsuccessful. The fragment extracted after removal of a bucket handle tear should be about 4 cm long.

Flap Tear

The same rules that were outlined for the longitudinal tear apply for the resection of a flap tear (Figs. **77** and **78**). The freely moveable part should initially be fixed with a needle. Thereafter the tissue bridge is cut from an ipsilateral or superior contralateral approach with a basket forceps or scissors until only a narrow bridge is left. After removal of

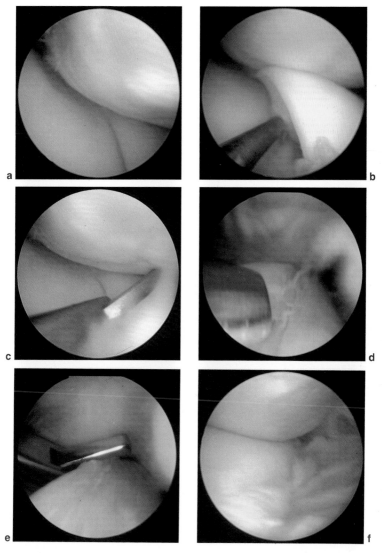

Fig. **75** Resection of a bucket handle tear in six steps. Arthroscopic photographs and schematic drawings. After repositioning, the bucket handle tear is to be treated like a simple longitudinal tear!

a overview
b diagnosis or repositioning
c resection of posterior horn
d grasping under tension
e resection of posterior horn
f examination after extraction

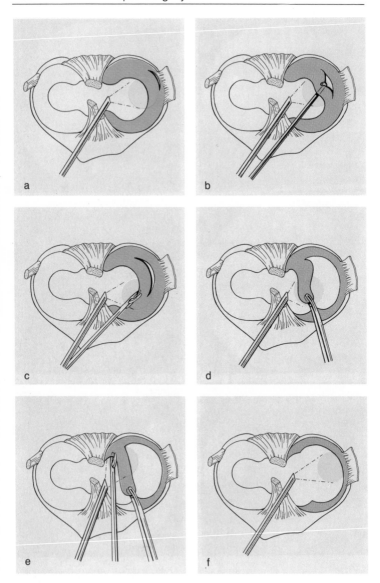

Fig. **76**   Schematic representation of the resection of a bucket handle tear in six steps corresponding to Figure **75**

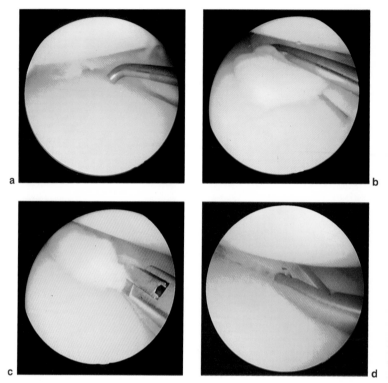

Fig. 77   Resection of a flap tear in four steps
a overview
b demonstration
c resection with remaining tissue bridge
d trimming after extraction

the fixing needle, the loose fragment is then extracted through the
dilated channel from the ipsilateral side. Further smoothing with the
90°-angled basket forceps may be necessary. Flap tears that are displaced posteromedially or posterolaterally should be repositioned and
then fixed with a needle. If this is unsuccessful, the resection should be
done in the posteromedial or posterolateral compartment through the
same approach. For this procedure, the arthroscope is advanced into the
appropriate compartment and the 70° scope is used. The knee is then
flexed 90°. To fully expand the posterior capsule, the intra-articular

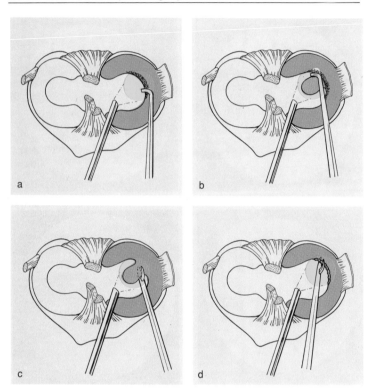

Fig. **78**   Resection of a flap tear in four steps corresponding to Figure **77**

pressure is elevated. Location of the posterior portal for instruments is facilitated by inserting a fine needle into the joint to check for the correct direction. The portal is enlarged with a sharp or blunt trocar, to allow introduction of surgical instruments. In most cases, a straight basket forceps is sufficient for the resection. For removal of the resected part of the meniscus, a large and strong grasping forceps is used (see also p. 113). The danger of losing parts of the meniscus during the course of their extraction through the different tissue layers should not be underestimated.

A similar procedure is used to remove fragments lost in the posterolateral or posteromedial compartments after resection of bucket handle tears.

Radial Tear

A radial tear can be resected with the basket forceps alone. In the region of the anterior horn, the resection is performed with the straight basket forceps from an ipsilateral approach while in the region of the posterior horn, a 90°-angled forceps is generally used. If the tear is far anterior, the instrument can be introduced from a contralateral approach to facilitate the resection. It is important to leave a smooth edge behind to avoid the risk of future ruptures (Fig. **79**).

The resection technique for both meniscus horns is similar to the resection of the ragged edges that routinely result from the resection of damaged parts of the menisci (Fig. **80**). The rough edge of the meniscus

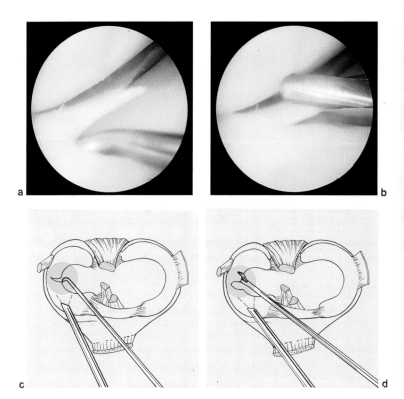

Fig. **79**   Trimming for radial tear. A radial tear is most commonly located in the middle third of the meniscus. Access is either through a high contralateral approach with a straight instrument or ipsilaterally with a 90°-angled instrument

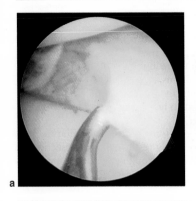

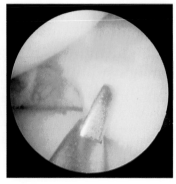

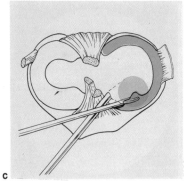

Fig. **80** After resection of the damaged parts of the meniscus, the ragged edges in the anterior part are trimmed with the 90°-angled basket forceps. Through a high contralateral approach a straight instrument can be used alternatively

is resected through a parallel approach with a 90°-angled instrument or through a high contralateral approach with a straight instrument.

Horizontal Tears

A horizontal tear is routinely associated with degenerative changes of the meniscus. Horizontal and so-called degenerative meniscus tears are therefore treated in the same manner. In most of these cases, significant tissue resection is required.

The most frequently used instrument is the basket forceps. For resection of a posterior horn tear, a straight basket forceps is introduced from an ipsilateral approach; in a tight knee, a straight 20° upward-curved basket forceps can be used to resect the destroyed posterior horn in its entirety (Figs. **81, 82**). The newly developed straight basket forceps with a broad cutting edge can shorten the time required for resection of a

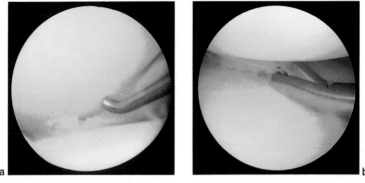

Fig. 81   Resection of a degenerative posterior horn with (**a**) a straight basket forceps and (**b**) with a basket forceps with an upward-curved tip

horizontal tear. Once the posterior horn is sufficiently trimmed, a 90°-angled basket forceps is introduced from an ipsilateral approach and the middle part of the destroyed meniscus is resected. Extensive use of the probing hook is necessary to determine the necessity and extent of the resection. The meniscus tissue is usually of poor quality and resection must be carried out close to the capsule to obtain a healthy tissue margin. It is the goal of the procedure to achieve a smooth transition to the anterior horn. Only healthy meniscus tissue should be left in the joint to avoid future tears. In general, an aggressive resection of degenerative meniscus tears is better than a conservative one.

If the horizontal tear is associated with a meniscus cyst, extensive resection and opening of the cyst region are necessary.

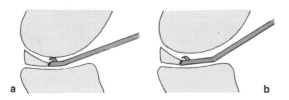

Fig. **82**   The schematic drawing shows that the shape of the selected instrument depends on the situation in the area of the posterior horn and on the shape of the femoral condyle. Instruments with an upward curve have proved particularly suitable

In most cases, an open surgical procedure can be avoided. Sometimes the exact location of the cyst cannot be determined during the first examination and palpation. In these cases, a needle placed from outside through both cyst and meniscus is helpful. Once the meniscus is resected in this area, the communication with the cyst becomes obvious. During the resection of a lateral meniscus in association with a cyst, a tissue bridge should be preserved over the popliteal tendon.

Large horizontal tears lend themselves to the use of powered tools for the resection. All unstable parts have to be removed. The rate of future ruptures should be under 1% if the resection was carried out into healthy tissue.

Discoid Meniscus

If a discoid meniscus is incidentally found without causing any symptoms, it does not need to be resected. If, however, a discoid meniscus is found that is of pathological significance (Fig. **83**) and might explain knee symptoms, it should be removed. The goal should be to preserve a residual meniscus similar to a normal-shaped meniscus after the resection. In the anterior horn, the redundant tissue can be resected with a straight knife from a superior contralateral approach. This fragment can then be extracted through the same channel with the grasping forceps after it is completely mobilized with the same straight knife. The remaining redundant tissue in the middle and posterior parts as well as rough edges can be resected and smoothed with the straight or the 90°-angled basket forceps. If available, powered tools can be helpful during these often extensive resections, provided the surgeon has the necessary experience.

Meniscus Repair

Indications for the Various Methods

Acute or old ruptures of variable length close to the capsule should be repaired if the tissue of the meniscus is of good quality. In the anterior and middle thirds, a direct arthroscopic suture can be performed, whereas in the posterior horn, an open surgical procedure is to be preferred since ruptures in this area often cannot be visualized well enough and the close proximity of nerves and blood vessels represents a constant risk during the arthroscopic procedure.

The central area of the meniscus is not vascularized. An indication for repair of a rupture exists therefore in the case of a bucket handle tear close to the base of the meniscus and of a tear through the area of vascularization, under consideration of the anatomical situation (Fig. **84**). After the diagnosis is established and the decision is made to attempt repair, a closed or open surgical procedure is planned. If the

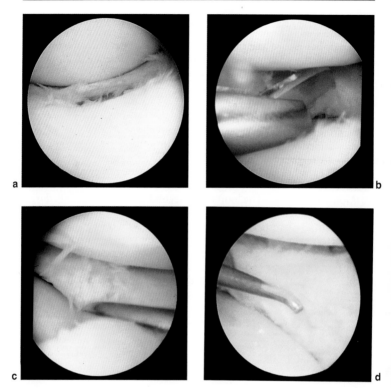

Fig. **83**   Resection of a discoid meniscus. The resection of a discoid meniscus using arthroscopic techniques has to be done in several steps because of the amount of tissue to be removed. Different techniques and instruments (shaver, electric knife) can be used

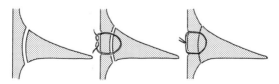

Fig. **84**   Schematic drawing of a meniscus repair. The suture should enclose the poorly vascularized part of the meniscus and connect it, "watertight", to the capsule. Very little or no suture material should traverse the joint space

surgeon is not well experienced in arthroscopic surgery, the open procedure should be preferred in every case. As the period of time until the repair has healed and the knee can bear weight is the same for both procedures, the patient has no disadvantages from the standpoint of recovery by having an open rather than a closed repair.

Arthroscopic Meniscus Repair

The repair is started at the anterior aspect of the tear after the repositioning of the fragment. After palpation of the jointline, two needles armed with 1–0 PDS sutures are introduced into the joint from outside through skin, capsule and meniscus and are placed about 3–5 mm central to the tear through the upper side of the meniscus. To facilitate the penetration with the needles, the meniscus can be held in position with a hook. The loop of the second needle is then pulled with the hook through the loop of the first needle and the first needle is withdrawn. The suture from the second needle is thereby brought out of the joint. Thereafter, both needles can be removed. This completes the first suture and the one end of the thread can now be brought subcutaneously to the other end to allow both ends to exit through one hole. In this fashion as many sutures are placed as necessary, usually three to five, and are tied subcutaneously under arthroscopic control (Fig. **85**).

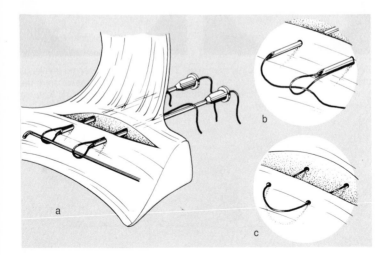

Fig. **85** Meniscus repair according to Gillquist. The torn fragment is adapted to the meniscus base by means of a U-shaped suture; this is done with two injection needles containing suture material (outside–in technique)

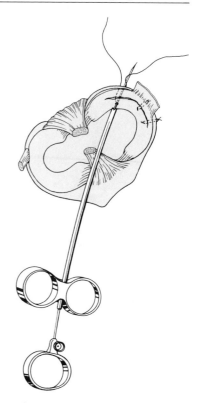

Fig. 86 Meniscus repair according
to Jakob. This technique utilizes a
double lumen guide instrument. Two
straight needles which are connected by a suture are passed through
this instrument to adapt the torn
fragment of the mensicus to its base
and then tie the two sutures in the
subcutaneous tissue after incision of
the skin (inside–out technique)

Another technique was described by Jacob. With the help of a guiding
instrument, two straight needles armed with an absorbable suture are
passed through both parts of the meniscus and are tied subcutaneously
on the outside after an incision has been made down to but not into the
capsule (Fig. **86**).

Open Meniscus Repair

The knee is positioned in 90° of flexion, either hanging down or in a
figure four position. A straight vertical incision of about 5 cm in length
is made along the posterior edge of the femoral condyle and the capsule
is incised (Fig. **87**). Medially, a capsular incision is made at the posterior
edge of the posterior oblique ligament and laterally at the posterior edge
of the lateral collateral ligament. Care must be taken not to injure the
saphenous nerve and vein medially or the peroneal nerve laterally. The

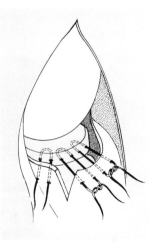

Fig. **87**   Open meniscus repair. To repair a meniscus torn close to its base, the suture should grasp a significant amount of tissue and should be tied outside the capsule without the suture material passing through the joint space. A row of sutures is placed from one end of the tear to the other. To facilitate repair, the meniscus base close to the capsule may be notched in the direction of the ligament fibers

intact junction between capsule and meniscus is incised vertically and the tear is inspected carefully (caution: semimembranous tendon). If the tear is old, the edges should be debrided with a sharp curette. Thereafter, the sutures are placed starting from the posterior. 2–0 Vicryl (polyglactin 910) on a curved needle is the preferred suture material. Several sutures are placed through the capsule, the meniscus, then back through the capsule in a vertical direction, and finally all sutures are tied. The incised junction between capsule and meniscus has to be closed with two separate sutures at the end.

A meniscus tear close to the capsule is commonly associated with a ruptured anterior cruciate ligament. Experience has shown that simultaneous reconstruction of the anterior cruciate ligament is advisable to diminish the risk for reruptures of the repaired meniscus.

Rehabilitation after Meniscus Repair

After meniscus repair, the knee is immobilized for four weeks in a long leg plastic splint in a position of 20° of flexion. Knee flexor and extensor muscles are exercised without weight-bearing through a range of motion from 20–60°. After four to six weeks, functional rehabilitation out of the posterior splint is started. Light exercises (bicycle riding, for example) can be started at 12 weeks, resistive range of motion exercises not before 16 weeks. The rehabilitation plan is similar for both arthroscopic and open meniscus repair.

Posterior Joint Space

Meniscus tears and loose bodies in the posterior compartments occasionally require open surgical treatment.

Loose bodies may be relatively large and cannot be brought into the anterior compartment, while smaller objects can be retrieved with the suction device and be maneuvered into the anterior joint space. If this is not possible, the extraction has to be done with a grasping forceps introduced from a posterior portal. Occasionally this is complicated by the fact that the irrigation fluid washes the object away from the forceps. Under these circumstances, the irrigation should be stopped

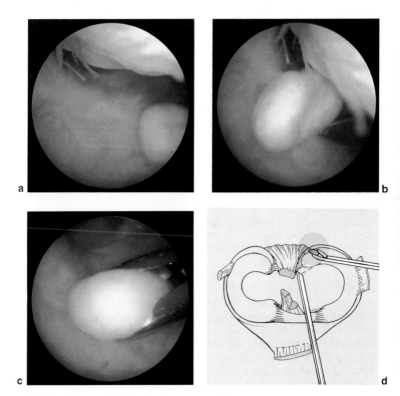

Fig. **88** A loose body in the posteromedial compartment of the knee joint is located (**a**) and the approach is determined using a wire or a cannula (**b**). Thereafter, a grasping instrument is introduced and the object is extracted through the capsule (**c**)

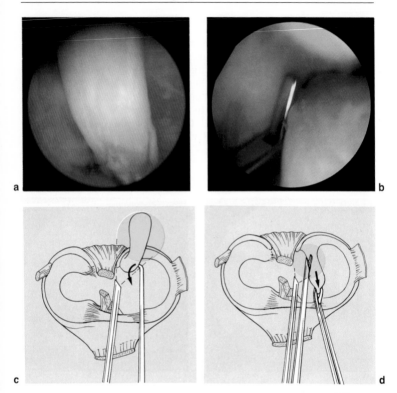

Fig. **89**   Resection of a meniscus flap folded over superiorly into the posterior compartment. The procedure is similar to the resection of a flap tear. If necessary, the fragment is removed through a posterior approach

and the loose body be brought by external movements into the reach of the grasping instrument. If this is not feasible, the suction device can be connected to the arthroscope and the object be brought closer to the forceps. Only when the loose body is securely held with the forceps should the exit channel be enlarged with the knife and the object pulled out (Fig. **88**).

Most meniscus tears can be treated from an anterior approach. Occasionally a posterior flap, however, is located high in the posteromedial compartment and is not accessible from any of the anterior portals. A bucket handle tear can also be dislocated in such a fashion and can disappear into the posterior compartment, particularly after it is transected at the anterior attachment or as a completely separated fragment.

In such cases, the posterior horn is separated through a paracentral approach, and the entire fragment is pushed back to be extirpated from a posterior portal. All tears in the posterior compartment represent some form of a flap tear and are treated in this fashion. The base of the meniscus is then usually close to the posterior cruciate ligament. Scissors or bucket handle forceps are introduced through a paracentral portal and allow the surgeon to cut the base of the meniscus under direct vision with the 30° scope (Fig. **89**). The remainder of the procedure is similar to that used for extraction of a loose body.

Lost Fragment

Occasionally the resected part of the meniscus cannot be retrieved or extracted. The further procedure depends on the situation and the location of the lost fragment.
The lost fragment could be:

— suprapatellar,
— parafemoral,
— in the posterior recess,
— in the soft tissues,
— in the drapes, towels, or sponges.

If the fragment could not be grasped initially it should be looked for in the joint space. The scope is placed in the intercondylar notch, all instruments are removed, and the joint is moved with near maximal distension. The search is started depending on accessibility in the superior recess, the medial and lateral recess, and in the posterior compartments. If the fragment was lost during the passage through the capsule the incision site should be digitally palpated and the fragment removed if present in the subcutaneous tissue layers. Occasionally the fragment is pushed out of the joint space by the intra-articular pressure and then can be found in the drapes, towels, or sponges.

Summary of Important Steps in Meniscus Surgery

Diagnostic evaluation is mandatory before starting any surgical procedure. The first decision is whether the meniscus should be preserved or resected. If a resection is to be performed, the easiest procedure should be chosen. The surgical strategy has to be outlined before the operation is started and should be followed step by step. If it does not lead to success, another plan should be made, but frequent changes of plans and approaches usually do not result in surgical success. Before the instruments are introduced into the joint space, the part of the meniscus that will be resected should be clearly visible since blind cutting only rarely leads to success. Occasionally orientation is disturbed by synovitis and a partial synovectomy is indicated in such cases. If the meniscus is severely damaged or if both menisci are damaged with degeneration of the cartilage and synovitis a powered tool should be used to shorten the operating time. An arthroscopic operation with preceding diagnostic arthroscopy should, in general, not take longer than one hour. Loose fragments, a resected part of the meniscus, for example, or other loose or foreign bodies should be removed in any case since they may cause blockage of the joint or synovitis. If the resection appears to be very difficult or the initial strategy does not lead to success within 45 min, a small arthrotomy should be performed without hesitation to resect the meniscus. A short arthrotomy is less traumatic for the patient than a prolonged arthroscopy with soft tissue edema and prolonged tourniquet application.

Some meniscus tears should be left alone. These are:

1. Short longitudinal tears (≤ 1 cm) close to the base if the meniscus is otherwise intact and not dislocated.
2. Short radial tears involving less than one third of the breadth of the meniscus.
3. Fresh tears close to the capsule in the vascularized part of the lateral meniscus (hiatus popliteus) without tendency to luxation.

During each meniscus resection, the joint should be irrigated and suctioned, particularly if a basket forceps is used. After the arthroscopic resection, a suction device has to be used to remove small fragments or debris. The suction should be activated intermittently to avoid blockage of the opening with synovial folds. If a pump is used, maximal irrigation should be used during this phase. Finally, the remaining meniscus is examined with the probing hook for stability.

Surgery of the Joint Surfaces

Arthroscopy is an excellent diagnostic tool for the joint surfaces, but the deeper layers cannot be evaluated. Similarly, arthroscopic surgery can only be applied to the superficial cartilage layers. Besides the diseases of the meniscus, diseases of the articular cartilage and the synovium are of interest. Under certain circumstances, even bone is visible and accessible. The main advantage of arthroscopy is the large area that can be visualized as compared with arthrotomy; the disadvantage is the difficulty in introducing second and third instruments into the joint through the different tissue layers.

Surgery of the Cartilage

The term chondropathy describes a mostly invisible pain phenomenon of the cartilage while chondromalacia refers to visible damage of the cartilage at different stages of severity. Surgical intervention cannot heal either of these conditions but may provide conditions that allow for faster healing.

If the chondromalacia is rather severe (Fig. **90**), the cartilage can be smoothed during arthroscopy. This can be done using hand instruments like curretes or, for larger areas, powered tools (Fig. **91**). Resection of the damaged cartilage into healthy tissue forms a good basis for further treatment. However, it is not clear whether these procedures routinely lead to the desired success.

Chondropathia patellae is a phenomenon consisting of a lateralization of the patella with pain during pressure and movement in which no or only minimal damage of the cartilage can be detected. The most prominent feature is a lateralized obliquely positioned patella. The procedure of choice is a lateral retinacular release, which can be performed both from the outside or arthroscopically. Using electro-resection, the lateral retinaculum of the patella can be resected together with the synovium. Using appropriate scissors, a lateral release (Fig. **92**) can be performed either subsynovially or under direct palpating control

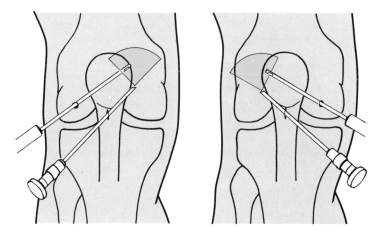

Fig. **90** Soft or detached pieces of cartilage are trimmed or resected. Hand instruments are useful to remove smaller pieces; the shaver should be used for larger areas. By using parallel procedures, only three portals are required in most cases

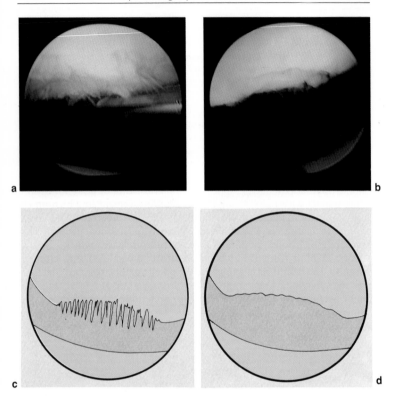

Fig. **91** Chondroplasty of the patella.
a Ragged cartilage before shaving
b After the procedure, the undersurface of the patella is smooth. Corresponding schematic drawings (**c**, **d**)

through the skin which results in improved gliding characteristics of the patella.

Surgery of the Bone

If the damage of the cartilage extends into the bone, Pridie drilling can be performed arthroscopically (Fig. **93**). For this purpose, a small drill or a wire is used and, after placement of a second or multiple incisions, the sclerotic cortical bone is opened. It is assumed that the presence of blood vessels allows for the formation of a good connective tissue bed

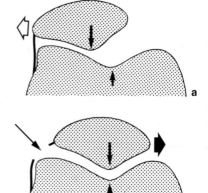

Fig. 92   Lateral release. Subluxation and lateralization of the patella are signs that the tension of the lateral retinaculum is excessive. This can be resolved by dividing these structures arthroscopically (**a**). The electrical resection knife can also be used for this purpose (**b**)

for the later formation of replacement cartilage, although exact studies of this problem are lacking.

The value of the surgery for so-called activated degenerative arthritis of the knee is doubtful. In our own experience good results have been achieved in some cases while it is not clear whether the surgical intervention, the subsequent drug therapy, or the rehabilitation were responsible for the improvement. In this particular procedure, the joint debris is removed through suction devices. Loose cartilage is removed, and osteophytes are resected. The elimination of rubbing and irritating particles inside the joint usually results in rapid and undeniable improvement. Appropriate rehabilitation is an integral part of this procedure.

If all these efforts fail in cases of severe osteochondral damage, or if diagnostic arthroscopy reveals such extensive damage that arthroscopic surgery does not seem appropriate, the arthroscopic examination is nevertheless still of value in determining wheter total joint replacement, osteotomies, or other joint preserving surgical procedures (for example, surgery according to Bandi or Maquet) should be performed.

On rare occasions, an arthroscopically controlled osteosynthesis of shearing fractures of the tibial plateau can be performed. The value of this method should not be overestimated, however. Extensive experience with open surgical procedures is required before one attempts arthroscopic osteosynthesis, as success is otherwise doubtful (Fig. **94**).

If routine radiological investigations have revealed the presence of osteochondritis dissecans, the loose fragment can often be fixed arthroscopically. In a well-equipped arthroscopy unit, the bed for the implant

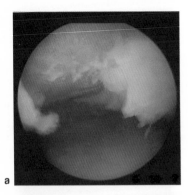

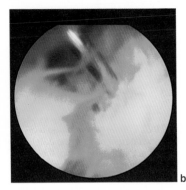

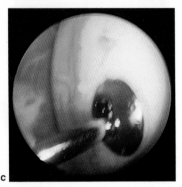

Fig. **93** Surgery of the bone. Advanced destruction of articular cartilage leads to an appearance somewhat comparable to "baldness" of the bone (**a**). Holes drilled deeply into the mostly ebonized bone reaching into the vascularized areas allow for the sprouting of connective tissue which forms tissue islands for subsequent formation of replacement cartilage (**b**). Small blood threads (in the picture) can be taken as a sign of successful opening of the sclerotic bone. Intra-articular osteosynthetic material can also be removed well by arthroscopy. The portal should be marked with a fine wire (**c**) before introduction of the grasping instruments or screw drivers

can be debrided appropriately before the fixation is attempted. For this fixation itself, osteosynthetic materials and Ethipins can be used.

Surgery of the Synovium

Synovitis resulting from other pathological conditions does not primarily require treatment during arthroscopy, but an improvement can be expected by just treating the underlying conditions.

If the synovitis represents an illness on its own, that is, chondromatosis synovialis or synovitis villonodularis, after confirmation by frozen section, a synovectomy must be performed.

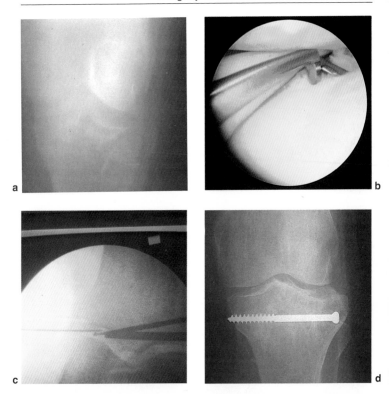

Fig. **94** Management of fractures. An avulsion fracture of the tibial plateau (**a**—tomogram) is confirmed arthroscopically (**b** probing hook and fixation wire). Under X-ray control (**c**), a compression screw is inserted parallel to the intra-articular wire with good reduction of the fracture (**d**)

This is, without doubt, a very difficult and lengthy procedure. The availability of sufficient irrigation and the appropriate equipment are prerequisites. The different types of files and cutters that can now be connected to a variety of suction devices and rotating instruments can be brought into almost any location within the joint and thus enable an arthroscopic subtotal synovectomy to be carried out. The posterior compartments which were not accessible for open surgical synovectomy even if two incisions were used should be included (Fig. **95**).

The plica synovialis mediopatellaris occasionally has clinical and pathological importance. Once other pathological conditions are excluded

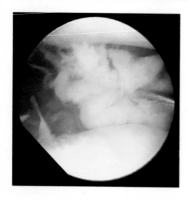

Fig. **95** Synovectomy. Arthroscopic synovectomy is very time consuming but clearly superior to open synovectomy

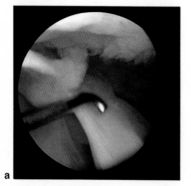
a

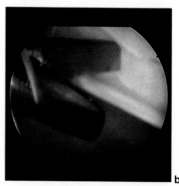
b

Fig. **96** Plica synovialis with pathological significance. (**2**) Splitting of a plica synovialis mediopatellaris hypertrophicans that had produced snapping and pain phenomena (**b**)

and the clinical impression and pathological appearance show it to be at fault, it should be removed. Only in rare cases does the contact area at the medial femoral condyle show chondromalacia; these circumstances are an unequivocal indication for its resection (Fig. **96**).

The plica can be incised and left in place or incised and removed via a high paracentral or suprapatellar approach. If flexion exercises are started early with an otherwise intact knee joint, the danger of a recurrent formation of fibrous bands is small. We prefer removal of the plica, as histopathological documentation is important.

Loose Bodies

Loose bodies appear in the joint space either primarily following chondromatosis or secondarily as a result of another traumatic or degenerative process. If they cause recurrent joint blockage, they must be considered freely mobile and should be removed (Fig. **97**).

The technique for removal of loose bodies depends on their size and number. If the loose bodies are rather small, they can be suctioned out through common suction devices. With repeated irrigation and suctioning, the joint can be completely emptied. If, however, the loose bodies are larger than the internal caliber of the suction device, grasping forceps should be used. Special instruments for extraction are also available. If necessary, the extraction channel has to be dilated. In all cases, the smallest loose body should be removed first, otherwise a large and undesired fluid leakage after extraction of the biggest loose body may make a continuation of the arthroscopy impossible.

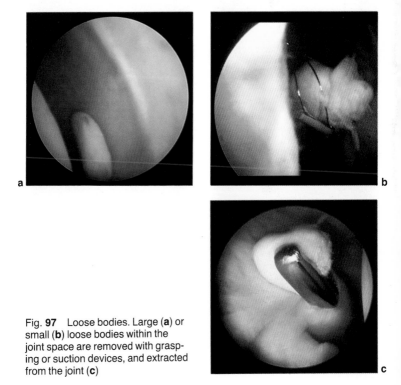

a
b
c

Fig. **97**   Loose bodies. Large (**a**) or small (**b**) loose bodies within the joint space are removed with grasping or suction devices, and extracted from the joint (**c**)

Arthroscopy and Miniarthrotomy

The term miniarthrotomy in connection with arthroscopy refers to an open surgical exploration of the joint using the smallest possible incision determined by preceding diagnostic arthroscopy (Fig. **98**).

In the early days of arthroscopy, proponents of arthrotomy held the opinion that a damaged meniscus would have to be completely removed to prevent future damage to the joint. While the arthroscopic removal of injured parts of the meniscus is a quick and relatively gentle proce-

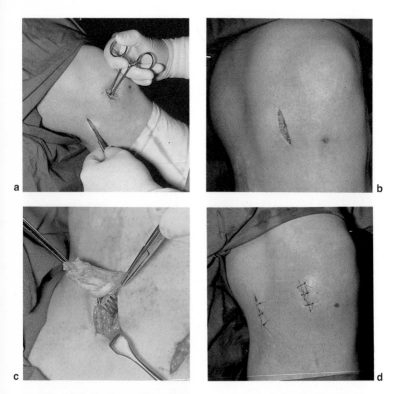

Fig. **98**   Miniarthrotomy. After arthroscopy, only the anterior attachment of the bucket handle tear could be resected from an anterior approach (**a**). The posterior margin of the medial collateral ligament is attached with a Kocher clamp (**b**). The posterior horn is divided and removed through a second small incision (**c**). The final result allows earlier rehabilitation than is possible after a conventional arthrotomy (**d**)

dure for the joint, the arthroscopic total meniscectomy has been associated with considerable difficulties. For some time, therefore, diagnostic arthroscopy was routinely followed by miniarthrotomy and total removal of the damaged meniscus using a small incision at an optimal site determined by arthroscopic examination. However, with the availability of more advanced instruments (suction forceps, powered tools, electrosurgery, etc.), total arthroscopic meniscectomy has become reality.

If, however, difficulties are encountered during arthroscopic surgery despite the use of second and third incisions to bring in additional instruments, one should not hesitate to switch over to an open procedure which then can be controlled arthroscopically. In most cases, this should be the least traumatic approach.

The site for the skin incision is determined arthroscopically and then marked with a needle. If the direction of the puncture is in alignment with the direction of the arthroscopic working instruments, a longitudinal incision is made, always taking the external structures of the joint into consideration. The damaged part of the meniscus is then exposed, using retractors and removed. In such cases, antibiotic prophylaxis is recommended and should be given intravenously before miniarthrotomy is started.

Replacement and Repair of the Cruciate Ligament

There is uniform agreement about the necessity to repair or replace the anterior curciate ligament, particularly in young and active patients, since the risks of recurrent problems and chronic instability of the joint are considered to be too high.

Since the late 1970s, therefore, any rupture of the anterior cruciate ligament, whether fresh or old, has been repaired surgically. Usually extensive open surgical procedures with inherent risks of traumatizing the joint were necessary and the thought of replacing these with arthroscopic procedures was appealing.

The possible surgical procedures include:

1. repair of the cruciate ligament; if necessary, with reinforcement,
2. autogenous reconstruction of the cruciate ligament,
3. prosthetic replacement of the cruciate ligament (Fig. **99a**),
4. combination of autogenous and prosthetic repair.

The repair of a cruciate ligament has rendered good results if the ligament had torn out at its insertion site with a bony fragment, thereby allowing refixation to the bone provided the ligament is not elongated. On the other hand, repairs of tears within the ligament itself have to be considered inadequate and weak if no additional reinforcement is used.

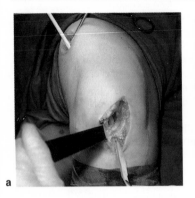
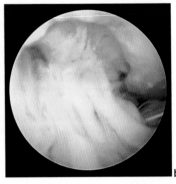

a   b

Fig. 99 Replacement of the cruciate ligament with an artificial prosthesis is almost completed after arthroscopic determination of the sites for the drill holes. Both ends are fixed to the bone with staples (**a**). One year after surgery, an arthroscopic check shows a well-functioning implant covered with synovium (**b**)

Attempts at arthroscopic repair of an intra-articular tear within the ligament itself are therefore unrealistic.

A reconstruction of the ligament with autogenous material is widely used today. The patellar tendon is used most commonly, and parts of it are redirected or repositioned. This procedure has the disadvantage of prolonged morbidity but usually renders good results (Fig. **99b**).

The anterior cruciate ligament can be completely replaced with synthetic material. The goal is to fix the graft to the bone in such a fashion that it exactly mimics the original ligament in its length, tension, and insertion sites. Procedures which use both autogenous and prosthetic material to replace the ligament should be called "hybrid" techniques. They combine early mobilization and stability with the advantages of longevity and a tendency for good healing offered by the autogenous material.

Various manufacturers offer different synthetic materials that have already been used in cardiovascular surgery for some time. The arthroscopic procedure to replace a cruciate ligament requires two additional incisions at the transition of the lateral femoral condyle to the shaft of the femur and at the medial side of the tibia. Both incisions have to be cut down to the bone. At these points that mark the insertion sites of the ligaments, holes are drilled into the bone under arthroscopic control. Although this is a proven and routine procedure nowadays with the advantages of early stability, mobility, a short hospitalization, and short morbidity, the fact that foreign material with its limited life expectancy is implanted in mostly young patients is of concern.

Different approaches to using autogenous material from different sites of the body are currently being evaluated.

Documentation, Rehabilitation, and Late Results

Documentation

Arthroscopy is a surgical procedure with opening of a joint cavity. Careful documentation is therefore mandatory in the patient's and the physician's interest. Videotaping of the procedure seems to be ideally suited to fulfill this requirement, as arthroscopy is done using optical instruments and is usually observed on a TV screen using a chip camera attached to the scope. These surgical documents have been found to be valuable for scientific as well as teaching purposes. The use of a 35 mm camera connected via an adapter to the scope allows at the same time photo documentation of the procedure. The intraoperative pictures in most textbooks of arthroscopy have been obtained using this technique. In clinical practice, however, still photography is only of limited value. A combination of written documentation and videotaping is ideally suited to allow the attending physician to interpret the intraoperative findings. A protocol has been developed combining schematic drawings, standardized notes, and free text that allows rapid interpretation, self-checking for the surgeon, and clear documentation of the findings in a simple form (Fig. **100**). This protocol has been used in Linköping since 1977 and has been found very valuable over a long period of time.

For the referring physician, two aspects of the documentation are of particular importance in the further care of a patient who has undergone diagnostic or surgical arthroscopy:

1. The result of the arthroscopy should be available, including history and physical examination.
2. Conclusions regarding short, middle, and long term rehabilitation that were drawn by the surgeon based on his or her findings and experience should be documented.

Written reports are suited particularly well to recommending rehabilitation protocols and to the reporting of preoperative physical findings. It is, however, difficult to report the arthroscopic intraoperative findings, and in our experience, a combination of schematic and optical documentation is much more valuable than a single still photograph of the joint.

Newer techniques allow documentation of the entire examination or operation or both, which is invaluable in teaching and in the improvement of methodology. Although such tapes or even the viewing of the procedure itself by the patient are offered by some institutions, the patient is usually not able to interpret the findings and their implications and still has to rely on the expertise of the physician.

The arthroscopic picture transferred from the scope to a TV screen can also be printed out directly on a connected printer, thereby allowing one to document the situation before and after certain procedures.

Another problem is the completeness of the documentation. Structures and areas that are not visualized should be specifically mentioned in the protocol. Incomplete or incorrect reports lead to disappointed referring physicians and disturbed patients. On the other hand, even a very detailed written report cannot replace an arthroscopic image; therefore, the precise and critical report should at least be supplemented by drawings.

Rehabilitation

Rehabilitation after arthroscopy covers as wide a spectrum as arthroscopy itself. The intensity of the rehabilitation process depends on the findings and the procedures. For example, after diagnostic arthroscopy without any pathological findings, fewer measures are necessary than after arthroscopic surgery. However, the arthroscopic examination represents a trauma in and of itself (incision, immobilization, ischemia time) and requires some postoperative consideration as well as the treatment of the underlying condition leading to the procedure. All surgical procedures on the knee joint should be considered according to the criteria given in Table **9**, and patients should be assigned to the different phases.

Postoperative Care

After arthroscopy is completed, the incision is closed with single sutures or simply taped. If liquid media were used, the suture can be omitted since spontaneous closure will follow edematous sweeling of the tissues. In this case, the amount of scar tissue is minimal and the stiches do not have to be removed. Postoperative management is similar to open surgical procedures and includes monitoring of the site of the operation and of the vital signs, DVT prophylaxis, and no weight-bearing.

After purely diagnostic arthroscopy, the patient can usually leave the hospital on the same day or the next; after surgical arthroscopy, the patient can be discharged after several days. All patients are checked on the fourth postoperative day, the dressing is changed, the joint is examined for effusion, and the incision is inspected. Up to 5% effusions after diagnostic arthroscopy and 15% effusions after surgical arthroscopy for about two to six weeks after surgery are tolerable. After puncture and compression dressings, immobilization and intermittent

Arthroscopy Protocol

File

Patient name   ☐☐☐☐☐☐☐☐☐☐☐☐☐

First name   ☐☐☐☐☐☐☐☐☐☐☐☐☐

D.O.B.   ☐☐☐☐☐☐

D.O.S.   ☐☐☐☐☐☐

Surgeon   ☐☐☐☐☐☐☐☐☐☐☐☐

Sex   ♂   ♀

right ◯   left ◯

Fresh injury (< 2 weeks) ◯   Hemarthrosis ◯   Serous effusion ◯

Preoperative diagnosis:

Postoperative diagnosis:

Comments:

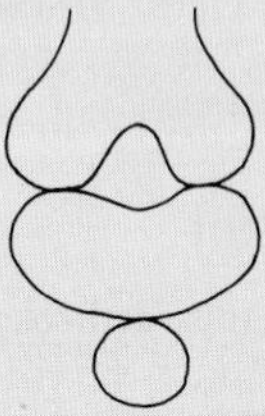

Technique	Instrument:	30° ◯		Access:	central ◯
		70° ◯			anterolateral ◯
	System:	Liquid ◯			anteromedial ◯
		Gas ◯			other ◯
	Bloodless field ◯			Local anesthesia ◯	
				Regional anesthesia ◯	
				General anesthesia ◯	

Findings

Medial meniscus	①	⓪	②	③	④	⑤	⑥	⑦	⑧	Cartilage, Femur medial	①	⓪	②	③	④
Lateral meniscus	①	⓪	②	③	④	⑤	⑥	⑦	⑧	Cartilage, Femur lateral	①	⓪	②	③	④
Medial ligament	①	⓪	②	③						Cartilage, Tibia medial	①	⓪	②	③	④
Anterior cruciate ligament	①	⓪	②	③	④	⑤	⑥			Cartilage, Tibia lateral	①	⓪	②	③	④
Posterior cruciate ligament	①	⓪	②	③	④	⑤	⑥			Popliteal tendon	①	⓪	②	③	
Patella	①	⓪	②	③	④					Synovia	①	⓪	②	③	
			⑤	⑥	⑦					Free body	◯				
										Chondromatosis	◯				
										Medial plica	◯				

Further treatment		**Arthroscopic surgery**	
Conservative	◯	Partial medial meniscectomy	◯
Arthroscopic surgery	◯	Total medial meniscectomy	◯
Arthrotomy	◯	Partial lateral meniscectomy	◯
		Total lateral meniscectomy	◯
		Incision of plica	◯
		Removal of free body	◯
		Pridie drilling	◯
		Biopsy	◯

Fig. **100** Our arthroscopy protocol with a combination of written and graphic descriptions. Front side (**a**)

Medial and lateral meniscus	0 not seen
	1 normal
	2 partially or totally removed
	3 radial tear
	4 horizontal tear
	5 longitudinal tear
	6 bucket handle tear
	7 flap tear
	8 degenerative
Medial ligament	0 not seen
	1 normal
	2 meniscofemoral ligament damaged
	3 meniscotibial ligament damaged
Cruciate ligaments	0 not seen
	1 normal
	2 partial rupture/elongation, old
	3 rupture, old
	4 partial rupture, fresh
	5 complete rupture, fresh
	6 s.p. ligament reconstruction
Patella	0 not seen
	1 normal
	2 chondromalacia I (softening)
	3 chondromalacia II (irregular surface)
	4 chondromalacia III (ulcer to the bone)
	5 subluxation I (disappears on flexion < 30°)
	6 subluxation II (disappears on flexion > 30°)
	7 subluxation III (remains during flexion)
Cartilage	0 not seen
	1 normal
	2 chondromalacia I (softening)
	3 chondromalacia II (irregular surface)
	4 chondromalacia III (ulcer to the bone)
Popliteal tendon	0 not seen
	1 normal
	2 rupture, old
	3 rupture, fresh
Synovia	0 not seen
	1 normal
	2 local synovitis
	3 generalized synovitis
Legend to illustrations	——————— Anatomical structure
	— — — — — Incision
	//////// Chrondromalacia I
	X X X X X Chrondromalacia II
	✸✸✸✸✸ Chrondromalacia III

b Reverse side with legend

Table **9** Phases of postoperative rehabilitation of the knee joint (after Zarins and Boyle)

Phase	Signs	Exercises
Immediate postoperative phase (Phase I)	fresh incision pain quadriceps weakness	quadriceps contraction straight leg raising possible external splint
Early healing phase (Phase II)	less pain 90° flexion quadriceps weakness effusion	isometric exercises bicycle exercises expanded range of motion
Late healing phase (Phase III)	no pain no significant weakness 120° flexion effusion possible	walking, bicycling, swimming isometric exercises
Rehabilitation and reconditioning (Phase IV)	full range of motion partial muscle rehabilitation limited sports activities no effusion	isokinetic exercises functional exercises stepwise increase in athlectic activities

use of ice packs for several days, repeated puncture is usually not necessary.

The phases in the healing process after arthroscopy and their associated phenomena have been summarized by Zarins (1985). All patients can be assigned their exercise and treatment regimens based on this classification. We offer a program for the routine work with postarthroscopy patients which is intended to offer some ideas and guidelines (pages 133–135). It should, however, be individualized for every patient.

Exercise Program after Operative Arthroscopy of the Knee Joint

This program is intended for knee joints with stable ligaments and disregards individual diagnoses. Attention is focused on the state of rehabilitation of the joint. The individual phases must be synchronized with the condition of the joint independent of time. The attending surgeon must state clearly whether treatment should be carried out in accordance with this program; if necessary, contraindications (bone or cartilage lesions, injuries of the ligaments, infection, etc.) must be pointed out together with instructions for changing the procedure. Maximum load is considered to be the weight load required for bending or stretching the knee 10 times.

Phase I (directly postoperative, even with drainage still in position)

1st exercise:
In supine position with knee supported; extend the knee (contract the quadriceps) 10 seconds per exercise, repeat about 10 to 15 times.

2nd exercise:
A flat pillow between both knees is compressed for about 10 seconds each time.

Phase I will usually last until the second postoperative day. It should be prolonged in case of exceptionally large swelling.

Phase II (initial healing phase)

3rd exercise:
In supine position, isometric contraction of the entire thigh musculature 10–15 times. Three series with a 15-second interval between them.

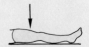

4th exercise:
In supine position; plant foot of the healthy leg on the table and move the extended operated leg up and down 10–15 times; 1–3 kg of weight can be added later. Three series with a rest period of 15 seconds between series.

5th exercise:
In supine position, extend the healthy leg and raise the extended operated leg and pull it inward and outward 5–10 times.

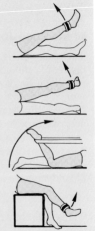

6th exercise:
In lateral position (on the healthy side), raise the extended operated leg for 10 seconds. Repeat about 10 times.

7th exercise:
In prone position, pull operated knee into flexion by means of a rubber band (Deuser band) for 10 seconds.

8th exercise:
Sitting on the edge of the table, bend and extend the knee with 1–3 kg of weight 10–15 times. Five series with a 20-second interval between them.

Phase II usually lasts up to the fourth postoperative day; depending on the type of surgery performed and on the condition of the knee, Phase II may even be prolonged to the tenth day.

Phase III (late healing phase)

9th exercise:
In supine position, the operated leg is held at approximately 30° of flexion and is raised and lowered 10–15 times, later with 1–3 kg of weight attached. Three series with 15-second intervals between them.

10th exercise:
In supine position, plant the foot of the healthy leg on the exercise table. With a roll placed under the operated knee, lift the extended leg approximately 10 cm off the support, hold for 10 seconds, repeat 10 times. Two series with 75% of maximal load; two-minute rest period between series.

11th exercise:
In lateral position (on the healthy side), raise and lower straight leg 10 times, later with 1–3 kg of weight. Three series with 15-second intervals between them.

12th exercise:
Sitting at the edge of the table, extend and flex the knee 20 times with 75% of the maximal load. Three to four series with 30-second intervals, between them.

13th exercise:
In a standing position with an ankle weight, bend
operated knee to 90° for 10 seconds 10–15 times
with 75% of the maximal load; two series.

Phase III can normally be started on the fifth day. It usually lasts until
the 20th day; this is followed by transition to isokinetic and functional
exercises, then advance to light sports activities.

Phase IV (rehabilitation and conditioning)

Transition to sports activities will succeed only through a combined
program of stretching and strengthening exercises.

Isometric Exercises:
14th exercise:
Downhill-skiing position; bend knees 30–60°; maintain this position for 30–60 seconds. Six series, repeat
twice with a two-minute interval between them.

15th exercise:
Stand on the operated leg bent between 30 and 80°,
swing the other leg in a circle rapidly with a slightly
bent knee 30–60 seconds, six series, repeat twice, two
minute interval between series.

Jogging: A distance of medium length should be covered several times
per week. Jog in a relaxed fashion and without ambition with respect to
duration and speed; good running shoes should be worn. Do not jog or
run on a hard surface!

Cycling: Cycle twice daily for 10–15 minutes on flat ground. Pay
attention to the correct height of the saddle (10° knee bend with lowest
pedal position) and low gear (do not overestimate yourself).

Phase IV should be continued up to the sixth week, depending on the
individual patient and on the findings. This is the best time for medical
follow-up checking; if the course has been normal, this should be the
turning-point for the permission of sports activities. If necessary, exercises should be continued.

Late Results

In the course of follow-up it will be necessary to document the result and any tendency toward improvement or toward deterioration in the patients state of health.

During follow-up examination, attention is focused on pain, swelling, and effusion. The results of arthroscopy are also assessed by the patient, who can articulate his or her satisfaction by means of a combination of purely subjective parameters and the test results. To approximate this "true" result of the knee-joint intervention, it will be appropriate to use the Lysholm score (Fig. **101**). The 100 points that represent maximum success are largely patient-oriented and are especially suitable for long-term comparisons.

However, first definite statements on the results of arthroscopy can be made only after six weeks at the earliest; follow-up examination after 12 months is particularly apt for the purpose of self-checking.

Operative arthroscopy is now about 20 years old. However, the method has been applied on a larger scale only during the last five years or so. It is only recently that elderly patients are being routinely treated arthroscopically for degenerative conditions of the joints.

It is evident from this that the medium- and long-term consequences of arthroscopy are not yet fully known. Of course it is impressive to experience patients being able to move their knees freely just a few hours after surgical removal of a lesion of the posterior horn of the meniscus. Any possible late damage, however, cannot be assessed at the present.

It has been said that the surgical possibilities of arthroscopy develop more rapidly than the possibility to assess the value of the method by means of clinical follow-up data. Exactly the same reservation is true for all innovative and rapidly acting methods of surgery. It goes without saying that this does not imply any positive or negative valuation.

Every patient should be followed up and re-examined regularly to detect any negative sequels as early as possible. Trends, too, must be identified and acted upon whenever necessary.

However, a few statements can be made even now:

1. A well-conducted arthroscopic operation is far superior to well-conducted open surgery as far as short-term results are concerned.
2. The method of partial meniscectomy is a great step forward with regard to the biomechanical function of the meniscus remnant.
3. Unsatisfactory results due to lack of technical skill are associated with the development of the method and recur with every beginner who starts practicing this method.
4. Arthroscopy even with negative findings results in clinical improvement in many cases.

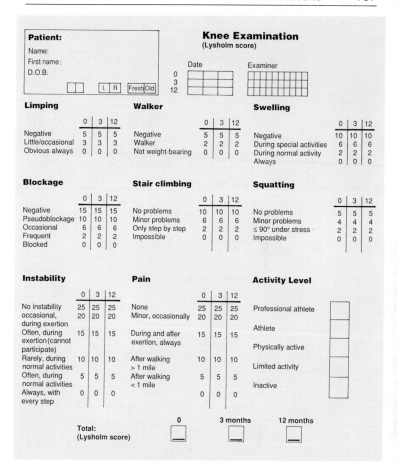

Fig. 101   Form for documenting knee examinations (after Lysholm)

5. Arthroscopic surgery of an activated arthrosis cannot be assessed with certainty at this time.

For a critical review of the late results of arthroscopy, it is imperative to refer to the original indication for the procedure. Late results will largely depend on the indication. Of course, a surgeon following severely restricted indication criteria will present less favorable results than a surgeon who practices arthroscopy on a liberal range of indications.

References

Basic Works

Chassaing V, Parier J. Arthroskopie des Kniegelenks. Cologne: Deutscher Ärzteverlag, 1988
Dandy D. Arthroscopy of the knee. London: Butterworth, 1984.
Glinz W. Diagnostische Arthroskopie und arthroskopische Operationen. Operationen am Kniegelenk. Berne: Huber, 1987.
Henche HR, Holder J. Die Arthroskopie des Kniegelenkes. Berlin: Springer, 1988.
Klein W, Huth F. Arthroskopie und Histologie von Kniegelenkserkrankungen. Stuttgart: Schattauer, 1980.
Shahriaree H, ed. O'Connor's textbook of arthroscopie surgery. Philadelphia: Lippincott, 1984.
Watanabe M. Arthroscopy of small joints. Tokyo: Igaku Shoin, 1985.

Journals

Arthroscopy: the journal of arthroscopic and related surgery. New York: Raven Press, 1985 – .
Arthroskopie: Organ der Deutschsprachigen Arbeitsgemeinschaft für Arthroskopie. Berlin: Springer, 1988 – .

Further Reading

Aigner R. Geräte für die Arthroskopie im Modulsystem. In Hefer H. Fortschritte der Arthroskopie. Stuttgart: Enke, 1985.
Alm A. The diagnostic value of arthroscopy of the knee joint. Injury 1974;5:319.
Apley G. The diagnosis of meniscus injuries: some new clinical methods. J Bone Joint Surg 1947;29 A:78.
Altmann RD, Gray R. Diagnostic and therapeutic use of the arthroscope in rheumatoid arthritis and osteoarthritis. J Am Med Assoc 1983;50.
Baker BE, Peckham AC, Pupparo F, Sanborn JC. Review of meniscal injury and associated sports. Am J Sports Med 1985;13:1.
Berner W, Tscherne H. Arthroskopische Diagnostik von Schultergelenksverletzungen. Unfallheilkd 1983:165.
Bircher E. Die Arthroendoskopie. Zentralbl Chir 1921;48:1460.
Blauth W, Donner K. Arthroskopie des Kniegelenkes. Stuttgart: Thieme, 1979.
Burman MS. Arthroscopy, or the direct visualization of joints: an experimental cadaver study. J Bone Joint Surg 1931;13:669.
Burman MS, Mayer L. Arthroscopic examination of the knee joint. Arch Surg 1936; 32:846.
Burman MS, Finkelstein H, Mayer L. Arthroscopy of the knee joint. J Bone Joint Surg 1934;16:255.
Casscells Sw. Arthroscopy: diagnostic and surgical practice. Philadelphia: Lea and Febiger, 1984.
Dandy DJ, Jackson RW. The impact of arthroscopy on the management of disorders of the knee. J Bone Joint Surg 1985;58 B:346.
Dandy DJ, Jackson RW. The diagnosis of problems after meniscectomy. J Bone Joint Surg 1975;58 B:349.
DeHaven KE. Diagnosis of acute knee injuries with hemarthrosis. Am J Sports Med 1980;8:9.
Delbarre F, Aignan M, Ghozlan R. L'arthroscopie du genou. Paris: Institut de Rhumatologie de la Faculté de Médecine, 1975.
Dick W, Glinz W, Henche HR, Ruckstuhl J, Wruhs O, Zollinger H. Kom-

plikationen der Arthroskopie. Arch Orthop Trauma Surg 1978;92:69.

Dorfmann H, Dreyfus P. Arthroscopy of the knee: methods and results. Minerva Med 1971;62:2621.

Dorfmann H, de Sèze S. Nouvelles observations sur l'arthroscopie du genou: résultat d'un expérience personelle. Semaine Hôp Paris 1972;48:3011.

Dorfmann H, Dreyfus P, Justin-Besançon, L. Arthroscopy of the knee joint: current status of the question. Semaine Hôp Paris 1970;46:3442.

Edgar MA, Lowy M. Arthroscopy ot the knee. Proc R Soc Med 1973;66:512.

Fick R. Handbuch der Anatomie und Mechanik der Gelenke, vol 1. Jena: Fischer, 1904:165.

Finkelstein H, Mayer L. The arthroscopy: a new method of examining joints. J Bone Joint Surg 1931;13:583−8.

Finochietto E. El signo del salto. Pern Med Argent 1930.

Flachenecker G, Fastenmeier K. Hochfrequenzgenerator mit automatischer Leistungsregelung für optimalen Schnitt. Urologe 1987;B27;1−4.

Fujimoto K. Arthroscopic findings of the experimental arthritis caused by intraocular injection of various disinfectant medicaments. Nippon Seikeigeka Gakka Zasshi 1949;22:60.

Gallannaugh S. Arthroscopy of the knee joint. Br Med J 1983;ii:285.

Geist EW. Arthroscopy: preliminary report. Lancet 1926;46:306.

Gillquist J. Operative arthroscopy. Endoscopy 1980;12:281.

Gillquist J, Hagberg G. A modified technique for arthroscopy of the knee. Acta Chir Scand 1976;142:123.

Gillquist J, Hagberg G. Findings at arthroscopy and arthrography in knee injuries. Acata Orthop Scand 1978;49:398.

Gillquist J, Hagberg G, Oretorp N. Arthroscopy in acute injuries of the knee joint. Acta Orthop Scand 1977;48:190.

Gillquist J, Hagberg G, Oretorp N. Therapeutic arthroscopy of the knee. Med. Diss. Nr. 57, Linköping, 1978:1−20.

Gillquist J, Hagberg G, Oretorp N. Arthroscopic examination of the posteromedial compartment of the knee joint. Int Orthop 1979;3:123.

Glinz W. Diagnostische Bedeutung der Arthroskopie bei Präarthrosen des Kniegelenkes. Unfallmed Berufskrankheiten 1984;4:260−5.

Glinz W. Die Arthroskopie bei Meniscusverletzungen. Unfallmed Berufskrankheiten 1976;3/4:106−15.

Glinz W. Arthroskopie beim Knorpelschaden des Kniegelenkes. Unfallheilkd 1976;127:46−57.

Glinz W. Arthroskopische Diagnostik der traumatischen Knorpelläsion im Kniegelenk. Unfallheilkd 1977; 129:242.

Glinz W. Diagnostische Arthroskopie und arthroskopische Operationen: Erfahrungen bei 500 Kniearthroskopien. Helv Chir Acta 1979;46:25.

Gminder F. Bestimmung der elektrischen Parameter bei der Hochfrequenzchirurgie [dissertation]. Munich: University of the Bundeswehr, 1987.

Hadied AM. An unusual complication of arthroscopy: a fistula between knee and the prepatellar bursa. J Bone Joint Surg 1984;66 A:624.

Hagberg G. On arthroscopy of the knee joints: a clinical study, with special reference to traumatic injuries [dissertation]. Linköping University, 1978.

Hamberg P, Gillquist J. Knee function after arthroscopy meniscectomy: a prospective study. Acta Orthop Scand 1984;55:172.

Hamberg P, Gillquist J, Lysholm H. A comparison between arthroscopic meniscectomy and modified open meniscectomy. J Bone Joint Surg 1984;66 B:189.

Hausmann B, Forst R. Nachweis einer möglichen Traumatisierung des Kniegelenkes bei der Arthroskopie. Z Orthop 1982;120:725.

Hempfling H. Farbatlas der Arthroskopie grosser Gelenke. Stuttgart: Fischer, 1987.

Henche HR. Indikation, Technik und Resultate der Arthroskopie nach Traumatisierung des Kniegelenks. Orthopäde 1974;3:128.

Henche HR. Indikation und Technik der Arthroskopie des Kniegelenkes. Orthop Prax 1976;2:165.

Henche HR. Die Arthroskopie des Kniegelenkes. Beitr Orthop Traumatol 1977;24:217.

Henderson CE, Hopson CN. Pneumoscrotum as a complication of arthroscopy. J Bone Joint Surg 1982; 64:1238.

Hertel P, Schweiberer L. Diagnostik der Meniskusläsion. Unfallheilkd 1981.

Hertz H. Arthroskopische Befunde bei frischen traumatischen Schulterluxationen und Konsequenz für die Therapie. Unfallheilkd 1983;165:167.

Holder J. Die arthroskopische Operation am Kniegelenk. Aktuel Traumatol 1982;12:222.

Hurter E. L'arthroscopie, une nouvelle méthode d'exploration du genou. Rev Chir Orthop 1955;41:763.

Ikeuchi H. Trial and error in the development of instruments for endoscopic knee surgery. Orthop Clin North Am 1982;13:263.

Imbert R. Arthroscopy of the knee: its technique. Marseille Chir 1956; 8:368.

Imbert R. Arthroscopy: significance of the method. Marseille Chir 1957; 9:676.

Ino S. Normal arthroscopic findings of the knee joint in adults. Nippon Seikeigaku Gakka Zasshi 1939;14:467.

Jackson RW. Arthroscopy of the knee. Curr Pract Orthop Surg 1973; 4:93−117.

Jackson RW. The role of arthroscopy in the management of the arthritic knee. Clin Orthop 1974;101:28−35.

Jackson RW. Diagnostic uses of arthroscopy. Recent Adv Orthop 1975;10:217−34.

Jackson RW. Current concepts review: arthroscopic surgery. J Bone Joint Surg 1983;65 A:416.

Jackson RW, Abe J. The role of arthroscopy in the management of disorders of the knee. J Bone Joint Surg 1972;54 B:310−22.

Jackson RW, Dandy DJ. Arthroscopy of the knee. New York: Grune and Stratton, 1976.

Jackson R, Haven EE De. Arthroscopy of the knee. Clin Orthop 1975;107.

Jackson RW, McCarthy DD. Arthroscopy of the knee. Toronto: University of Toronto Press, 1971:293−7.

Jäger M, Wirth CJ. Kapselbandläsionen. Stuttgart: Thieme, 1978.

Jakob RP, Stäubli HU. Indikation, instrumentelle Technik und Ergebnisse der arthroskopischen Meniskusrefixation. In: Hofer H, ed. Fortschritte in der Arthroskopie. Stuttgart: Enke, 1985:157.

James S. Surgical anatomy of the knee. Fortschr Med 1978;96:139.

Jayson MI. Arthroscopy: a new diagnostic method. Nurs Times 1968; 64:1002.

Jayson MI, Dixon ASJ. Arthroscopy of the knee in rheumatic diseases. Ann Rheum Dis 1968;27:503.

Jensen JE, Conn RR, Hazelrigg G, Hewegg JE. The use of transcutaneous neural stimulation and isokinetic testing in arthroscopic knee surgery. Am J Sports Med 1985;13:27.

Johnson LL. Diagnostic arthroscopy of the knee. In: International Congress on the Knee Joint. Rotterdam, 1973.

Johnson LL, Becker RL. The role of the assistant in arthroscopy. In: 42nd Annual Meeting of the American Academy of Orthopedic Surgeons, March 1985.

Johnson LL, Becker RL. Arthroscopy: technique and the role of the assistant. Orthop Rev 1976;9:31.

Johnson LL, Shneider DA, Becker RL. Arthroscopy 76. In: 43rd Annual Meeting of the American Academy of Orthopedic Surgeons, January-February 1976.

Kapandji IA. Funktionelle Anatomie der Gelenke, vol 2. Stuttgart: Enke, 1985.

Karpf MR, Aigner R, Gradinger R. Verletzungen des Kniegelenks. In: Lange M, Hipp E, eds. Lehrbuch für Orthopädie und Traumatologie, vol 3. Stuttgart: Enke, 1986.

Kawashima W. Arthroscopy of the tuberculous knee in its early stage. Nippon Seikeigeka Gakka Zasshi 1943;18:651.

Kieser C, Rüttimann A. Die Arthroskopie des Kniegelenkes. Schweiz Med Wochenschr 1976;106:1631.

Klein W, Schulitz KP. Arthroscopic meniscectomy. Arch Orthop Trauma Surg 1983;101:231.

Klose HH, Schuchardt E. Wertigkeit der Meniskuszeichen. Orthop Prax 1979.

Kohn D, Aigner R. Entscheidungen vor, während und nach der Kniegelenksarthroskopie. Fortschr Med 1985; 103:317.

Koike F. Arthroscopic study of experimental suppurative arthritis. Nippon Seikeigeka Gakka Zasshi 1943; 18:656.

Kolditz D, Krämer J, Eichhorn J. Die Technik der Elektroresektion bei arthroskopischen Kniegelenksoperationen. In: Hafer H, ed. Fortschritte in der Arthroskopie. Stuttgart: Enke, 1985:244.

Kreuscher P. Semilunar cartilage disease: a plea for early recognition by means of the arthroscope and early treatment of this condition. Illinois Med J 1925;47:290.

Kuner EH, Thürck HU, Lippe J von der. Zur Diagnostik und Therapie der akuten Kniegelenksinfektion. Unfallchirurgie 1987;13:249.

Lanz T von, Wachsmuth W. Praktische Anatomie, vol 1, part 3. Berlin: Springer, 1959.

Lesky E. Vom Lichtleiter zum Zystokop. Med Monatsspiegel 1966;4:76–80.

Lewicky RT, Abeshaus MM. Simplified technique for posterior knee arthroscopy. Am J Sports Med 1982;10:22.

Lidge RT. Problems and complications in arthroscopy. In: Casscells CS, ed. Arthroscopy: diagnostic and surgical practice. Philadelphia: Lea and Febiger, 1984.

Lindberg U. The patellofemoral pain syndrome [dissertation]. Linköping, 1986. (Medical dissertation 277.)

Lindenbaum BL. Complications of knee joint arthroscopy. Clin Orthop 1981;160:158.

Lipson RL, Clemmons JJ, Frymoyer JW. Arthroscopy experience with percutaneous biopsy of intra-articular structures under direct vision. Arthritis Rheum 1967;10:294.

Lundberg M, Odensten M, Hammer R, Hamberg P, Lysholm J, Gillquist J. Instruments for routine arthroscopic surgery of the knee. Acta Chir Scand 1984;520(suppl):79.

Lysholm J. Arthroscopy in surgery of the knee [dissertation]. Linköping, 1981. (Medical dissertation 106.)

Lysholm J, Gillquist J. Arthroscopic examination of the posterior cruciate ligament. J Bone Joint Surg 1981;63 A:363–6.

Lysholm J, Gillquist J. Endoscopic meniscectomy: follow-up study. Int Orthop 1981;5:265–70.

Lysholm J, Gillquist J, Liljedahl SO. Arthroscopy in the early diagnosis of injuries to the knee joint. Acta Orthop Scand 1981;52:111.

McGinty JB. Arthroscopic surgery update. Baltimore: University Park Press, 1985.

Mariani PP, Gillquist J. The blind spots in arthroscopic approaches. Int Orthop 1981;5:257.

Mariani PP, Gigli C, Puddu G, Ferretti A. Long-term assessment of negative arthroscopies. Arthroscopy 1987; 3:53.

Matsumo J. Arthroscopic and histologic studies of tuberculosis and nonspecific chronic arthritides. J Jap Assoc Rheum 1959;1:409.

Mayer L, Burman MS. Arthroscopy in the diagnosis of meniscal lesions of the knee joint. Am J Surg 1939;43:501.

Mennet P. Möglichkeiten und Grenzen der Kniearthroskopie. Schweiz Med Wochenschr 1974;101:1591.

Metcalf RW. Meniscectomy by triangulation through medial and lateral portals. In: Casscells SW, ed. Arthroscopy. Philadelphia: Lea and Febiger, 1984.

Müller W. Die verschiedenen Typen von Meniskusläsionen und ihre Entstehungsmechanismen. Unfallheilkd 1976;128:39.

Müller W. Das Knie. Form, Funktion und Ligamentäre Wiederherstellungschirurgie. Berlin: Springer, 1982.

Noble J, Hamblen DL. The pathology of the degenerative meniscus lesion. J Bone Joint Surg 1975;57B:180.

Noyes F, Basset RW, Grood ES, Butler DC. Arthroscopy in acute traumatic haemarthrosis of the knee. J Bone Joint Surg 1980;62A:687.

Noyes F, Spievack ES. Extra-articular fluid dissection in tissues during arthroscopy. Am J Sports Med 1982;10:346.

O'Connor RL. The arthroscope in the management of crystalinduced synovitis of the knee. J Bone Joint Surg 1973;55A:1443.

O'Connor RL. Arthroscopy in the diagnosis and treatment of acute ligament injuries of the knee. J Bone Joint Surg 1974;56A:333.

O'Connor RL, Salisburg RB, Shahriaree H. Synovial disease. In: Shahriahree H, ed. O'Connor's textbook of arthroscopic surgery. Philadelphia: Lippincott, 1984.

Ohnsorge J. Arthroskopie des Kniegelenkes mittels Glasfasern. Z Orthop 1969;106:535.

Okamura T. An arthroscopic study of the traumatic disorders of the knee joint. Nippon Seikeigaka Gakka Zasshi 1945;23:28.

Oretorp N. Anterior midline or central approach to arthroscopic meniscectomy. In: Casscells SW, ed. Arthroscopy: diagnostic and surgical practice. Philadelphia: Lea and Febiger, 1984:147.

Outerbridge RE. The etiology of chondromalacia patellae. J Bone Joint Surg 1961;43B:752.

Peek RD, Haynes DW. Compartment syndrome as a complication af arthroscopy: a case report and a study of interstitial pressures. Am J Sports Med 1984;12:464.

Pettrone FA. Meniscectomy: arthrotomy versus arthroscopy. Am J Sports Med 1982;10:355.

Robles Gil J, Katona G. Arthroscopy as a means of diagnosis and research: review of 80 arthroscopies. Amsterdam: Excerpta Medica, 1969. (Excerpta Medica international congress series, 209.)

Robles Gil J, Katona G. Clinical and therapeutic usefulness of arthroscopy. Gazzetta Sanit 1971;20:16.

Robles Gil J, Katona G, Barroso MR. Arthroscopy as an aid to diagnosis and investigation. Amsterdam: Excerpta Medica, 1968. (Excerpta Medica international congress series, 143).

Scharizer E. Fehler bei der Diagnose von Meniskusverletzungen. Unfallheilkd 1957;60:5.

Schonholtz GJ. Complications of arthroscopic surgery. In: Shahriahree H, ed. O'Connor's textbook of arthroscopic surgery. Philadelphia: Lippincott, 1984.

Schulitz LP, Huth F. "Plica-Krankheit" des Kniegelenkes. Dtsch Med Wochenschr 1979;104:1261−4.

Simonsen O, Jensen J, Moritzen P, Lauritzen J. The accuracy of clinical examination of injury of the knee joint. Injury 1984;16:96−101.

Simpson LA. Factors associated with poor results following arthroscopic subcutaneous lateral retinacular release. Clin Orthop 1984;186:165−71.

Sweeny HJ. Teaching arthroscopic surgery at the residency level. Orthop Clin North Am 1982;13:255.

Takagi K. The arthroscope. Nippon Seikeigaka Gakka Zasshi 1939;14:359−41.

Tesson MC, Aignan M, Delbarre F. Arthroscopy of the knee: technique, indications, results. Presse Méd 1970;78:2467.

Thorblad J, Ekstrand J, Hamberg P, Gillquist J. Muscle rehabilitation after arthroscopic meniscectomy with or without tourniquet control. Am J Sports Med 1985;13:133.

Toth S, Varsanyi Z. Über den diagnostischen Wert der Arthrographie mit positivem Kontrastmittel bei den Bandverletzungen des oberen Sprunggelenkes. Monatschr Unfallheilkd 1974; 77:543.

Trillat A. Les lésions méniscales internes. Rev Chir Orthop 1972;57:318.

Tsuyama N, Udagawa E. Arthroscopy. Surg Ther (Osaka) 1966;14:581.

Walker PS, Hajek J van. The loadbearing area in the knee joint. J Biomech 1972;5:581.

Watanabe M. The development and present status of the arthroscope. J Jap Med Inst 1954;25:11.

Watanabe M. Arthroscopy of the knee joint. In: Helfet AJ, ed. Disorders of the knee. Philadelphia: Lippincott, 1974:139.

Whipple TL, Bassett FH. Arthroscopic examination of the knee. J Bone Joint Surg 1978;60 Aß444.

Wredmark T, Lundh R. Arthroscopy under local anaesthesia using controlled pressure: irrigation with prilocaine. J Bone Joint Surg 1982;64 B:583.

Index

A

Air embolism, 25
Arcuate ligament, 12
Arthritis, active degenerative, surgery,
    119
Arthrography, and interval before
    arthroscopy, 75
Arthroscopy, diagnostic
  acute trauma, 93–97
  alternative methods, 59
  anesthesia, selection, 23–24
  approaches and maneuvers, 20,
    29–32, 60–64
    blind spots, 31
    design of approach, 65
    systematic step-by-step approach,
      71
  arthrotomy during same anesthesia,
    52–53
  contraindications, 58–59
  disorders of synovial membrane,
    91–92
  evaluation of articular cartilage,
    86–89
  evaluation of patella, 89–90
  examining the capsule and
    ligaments, 82–86
  examining the joint space, 64–74
  examining the menisci, 74–82
  filling medium
    gas insufflation, 24–25
    liquid media, 25–29
    selection, 24–29
  indications, 55–58, 60
    grouping by structures, 55
    step-by-step evaluation, 56
  informed consent, 48
  learning, step-by-step technique,
    2–3
  and miniarthrotomy, 124–125
  operative procedure, preparation
    and positioning, 48–50
  plica syndrome, 92–93
  prerequisites, 22

problems and complications,
    53–54
  procedure
    choice, 22–23
    completion, 51–52
  protocol and descriptions,
    130–131
  secondary procedure, delayed, 52
  selection of instruments, 32–42
  time for procedure, 52
  work place, 47
  see also Arthroscopy, surgical
Arthroscopy, diagnostic vs. surgical,
    23
Arthroscopy, surgical
  advantages over open surgery, 1–2
  approaches and maneuvers, choice
    of approach, 20, 29–32,
    60–64
  filling medium, 24–29
  informed consent, 48
  late results, 135–137
  problems and complications,
    53–54
  survey of indications, prerequisites
    and techniques, 98–99
  see also Arthroscopy, diagnostic;
    specific structures and condi-
    tions
Arthrotomy
  during same anesthesia, 52
  following arthroscopy, contraindi-
    cations, 52
Articular cartilage
  damage, 54
  evaluation, 86–89
  lesions, grading, 87–89
  pathological changes, 88
  surgery, 117–118

B

Biomechanics of the knee joint, 19–21
Bony structures of the knee
  anatomy, 7–10
  sagittal section, 5

C

Capsule, examination, 82–86
Cartilage *see* Articular cartilage
Chondromalacia, surgery, 117–118
Chondropathia patellae, surgery, 117–118
Compartment syndrome following arthroscopy, 94
Computed tomography, menisci, 75
Consent to arthroscopy, 48
Cruciate ligaments
  anatomy, 13–14
  anterior, rupture, 96
  arthroscopy, 84–85
  common synovial sheath, 6
  confusion with ligamentum mucosum, 7
  lesions, provocation tests, 96
  posterior, rupture, 96
  reconstruction with prosthesis, 126–127
  surgical procedures, 125–127

D

Documentation, 128–129
Drawer test
  anterior, posterior and Lachman, 82
  and contraindications to arthroscopy, 58

E

Effusions, postoperative, 129
Electroresection, 42–46
Eminentia intercondylaris, 8
Exercise program after operative arthroscopy, 132–135

F

Femoral axis, and tibial axis, malalignment in valgus deformity, 10
Femoral condyles, 68
Fibula fracture, contraindications to arthroscopy, 94
Fibular nerve, 19
Fluid media *see* Liquid media
Fractures
  contraindications to arthroscopy, 58
  fibula fracture, 94
  intercondylar eminence, 95
  tibial plateau, management, 121

G

Ganglions, hiatus popliteus, 15
Gas insufflation, 24–25
  contraindications, 45, 54
  leakage, 54
Gastrocnemius muscle, 12, 13
Generators used in electroresection, 42–46

H

Hemophilia, synovial damage, 92
Hiatus popliteus
  examination, 69
  normal view, 72
  preservation, 79
  and vascular supply to menisci, 15
Hoffa's fat pad, 5

I

Iliotibial band, 10
Infection, suspicion, post arthroscopy, 53
Instruments
  basic set, 40
  electroresection, 42–46
  hand instruments, 34–39
  maintenance and sterilization, 51
  optical and video systems, 32–34
  power systems, 39–42
  selection of instruments, 32–42

Intercondylar eminence, fracture, 95
Intercondylar notch, 68

J

Joint space
   anatomy, 4–7
   effusion and swelling, flexion position of joint, 6
   empyema, decompression and evacuation by arthroscopy, 53
   examination, 64–74
   lateral, 68–69
   lateral recess, 69
   loose bodies, 123
   medial, 68
   normal views by arthroscopy, 72–73
   plicae, 4–7
   posterior compartments, 69
   posterior space, loose bodies, 113–114
   subsynovial rupture, 84
   tamponade, 92
   volume, 5
Joint surfaces
   surgery of the bone, 118–120
   surgery of the cartilage, 117–118
   surgery of the synovium, 120–122
Juxta-articular structures, 18–19
   approaches and maneuvers, 20

L

Lachman test, 83
Leg position for operation, 48–50
Ligaments of the knee
   arcuate ligament, 12
   collateral ligaments, 84–86
      lateral side, 12, 13
      medial side, 11–12
      rupture, 96
   examination, 82–86
   "law of the ligaments," 4
   posterior aspect, 13
   treatment, 97
   see also Cruciate ligaments
Ligamentum mucosum
   anatomy, 4–7
   confusion with cruciate ligaments, 7
Liquid media, 25–29

characteristics, 28
fluid leak, 54
inflow cannula, 25–26
RPM-controlled pump, 26
in suspicion of infection, 53
Loose bodies, synovial space, 123
Lysholm Score, assessment of results of surgical arthroscopy, 136

M

Mechanics of the knee, 21
Medial collateral ligament see Ligaments
Menisci
   bilateral tears, 82
   biomechanics, 14
   bucket handle tear, 78
      resection, 100–102
   crash rupture, 97
   cysts, 79
   discoid meniscus, 79–82
      resection, 108–109
   examination, 74–82
   flap tears, 78
      resection, 100–104
   horizontal tears, 79
      associated with cyst, 107–108
      posterior horn, 106–107
      resection, 107–108
   lateral meniscus, 12
   longitudinal tear, 76–78
      undisplaced type, 99–100
   meniscectomy
      consequences, 17, 19
      follow-up, 17
      incidence, 74
      meniscus affected, 74–75
      sex of patient, 74
   normal function, 14–15, 18
   posterior compartment, tears and loose bodies, 113–115
   primary degenerative changes, 17
   radial tears, 79
      resection, 105–106
   repair
      direct suture by arthroscopy, 108–111
      lost fragments, 115
      open repair, 111–112
      rehabilitation following, 112

summary of important steps,
115–116
space-occupying effect, 15
symptoms of lesions, 75
tears
development, 74
diagnosis, 74–75
not needing repair, 116
types, location and examination,
75–82
vascular supply, 15–16
Miniarthrotomy, preceded by arthroscopy, 124–125
Muscles and ligaments
anterior side, 11
lateral side, 11

O

Operative procedure see Arthroscopy
Optical and video systems, 32–34
Osteochondral traumatic lesions, 95
Osteochondritis dissecans, indications
for arthroscopy, 56

P

Patella
acute dislocation, 95
chondropathia patellae, surgery,
117–118
evaluation, 89–90
and its mechanics, 9
osteochondral lesions, 95
patella baja, 58, 60
visualization, 72
patellar tendon, approach for
arthroscopy, 29–32, 60–64
Q-angle, 9
retinacula, 11, 119
suprapatellar recess, 65, 69
normal view, 72
underside, 65, 72
Peroneal nerve, 19
Pes anserinus, 12
"Pivot shift," tibial plateau, 10
Plica infrapatellaris, 5
Plica syndrome, 92–93
Plica synovialis mediopatellaris hypertrophicans, 122
Popliteal muscle, 12, 13

visualization, 72
Portals see Arthroscopy, diagnostic,
approaches and maneuvers
Postoperative care, 129–132
exercise program after operative
arthroscopy, 132–135
Power systems, 39–42
Pridie drilling, 118
Pumps for fluid irrigation media,
25–28
control of flow rate, 29
see also Liquid media

R

Radiographs, Frik's view, 8
References and further reading,
138–143
Rehabilitation, 129
exercise program after operative
arthroscopy, 132–135
phases, 132
Retinacula, patella, 11, 119
Rigidity ("tightness") of the knee, 71

S

Saphenous veins, 19, 20
Semimembranous muscle, 12
Synovial chondromatosis, 92
Synovial membrane, disorders, 91–92
Synovial space see Joint space
Synovitis, synovectomy, 120–122
Synovitis villonodularis, 91, 92

T

Tibial compartment syndrome, 19
Tibial plateau
anatomy, 6
avulsion fracture, 121
impression fracture, 95
"pivot shift," 10
shearing fractures, osteosynthesis,
119
Trauma, acute
diagnostic arthroscopy, 93–97
types, 95–97
Trochlear groove, 65

V

Valgus deformity, malalignment of
    femoral and tibial axis, 10
Varus and valgus stress tests, 82
Video, disinfection for operation, 51